بسم الله الرحمن الرحيم

Islamic Medicine
An Introduction

by

M. Salim Khan
M.D. (M.A.) M.H. D.O.

Mohsin Health
446 East Park Road, Leicester, LE5 5HH, UK
Telephone: +44 116 273 8614
Email: info@mohsinhealth.com

19 SHAWWAL 1444

10 MAY 2023 CE

This 6th expanded edition was published in May 2023

Published by: Mohsin Health
446 East Park Road, Leicester, LE5 5HH, UK
Website: www.mohsinhealth.com
E-mail: info@mohsinhealth.com

Disclaimer: This book is not intended to provide medical advice, diagnoses, or treatments, as it is for general information only. Always consult a qualified healthcare professional for your healthcare needs, and to advise you on what foods, activities, and treatments are suitable or unsuitable for you as an individual. The authors, editors, and publishers disclaim liability for any harm arising from the use of this book or any of its contents.

ISBN-13: 978-0-9929456-2-6

CONTENTS

INTRODUCTION 1

1. HISTORICAL BACKGROUND 2

Health and Medicine in Pre-Islamic Arabia 2

Medicine in the Early Period of Islam 7

The Umayyad Period 13

The Abbasid Period 16

Later Works 21

2. PHILOSOPHICAL CONCEPTIONS OF ISLAMIC MEDICINE 24

Ilm: the Light of True Knowledge 24

Islam: an Integrated Unity 27

Tawhīd: the First Principle and Methodology of Unification 28

The Human Being: a Microcosm 31

The Ḥakīm: a Symbol of Unity 33

3. THE PSYCHOLOGICAL FOUNDATIONS 34

The Human Being: an Integrated Whole 34

The Unity and Diversity of Nafs: the Self 35

The Origin and Functions of Rūḥ: the Vital Force 35

Aspects of Rūḥ 37

4. Physiological Concepts **41**
Arkān: the Elements 42
Akhlāt: the Humours 45
Mizāj: Temperament 48
Temperaments of the Organs 50
Temperaments of Medicines 51
Ā'dā': the Organs 52

5. Life Balance **56**
Ecological Considerations 57
Mental and Emotional Factors 60
Sleep and Wakefulness 61
Diet and Nutrition 61
Physiological Movement and Rest 63
Retention and Elimination 64

6. Diagnosis **65**
Indications of Health 65
Classifications of Disease 66
Signs of Temperaments 68
Pulse 71
Urine 74
Stool 76

7. PREVENTATIVE ASPECTS **78**
Personal Hygiene 78
Community Health Measures 86
Fasting: an Institution for Health Promotion 87

8. PRINCIPLES OF TREATMENT **89**
Management of Essential Factors 89
Treatment Through a Single Remedy 92
Use of Compound Medicines 95
Use of the Qur'an In Healing 97
Surgical Intervention 98

9. THE FUTURE OF ISLAMIC MEDICINE **100**
Socio-cultural Implications 100
Economic Considerations 102
Towards Health, Happiness and Peace 103

GLOSSARY **104**

NOTES AND REFERENCES **110**

SELECTED PROPHETIC RECIPES AND INGREDIENTS FOR MAINTAINING AND IMPROVING HEALTH AND WELLBEING **119**

INDEX **132**

Maps

Map 1: Pre-Islamic Arabia 3

Map 2: Arabia at the Time of Muhammad صلى الله عليه وسلم 11

Map 3: the Umayyad Period 15

Diagrams

Fig. 1: the Polarisation of Quwwah/Energy 41

Fig. 2: the Relative Positions of the Elements 44

Fig. 3: the Relationships of the Seasons, Elements and Humours 46

Fig. 4: Hierarchical Classification of Diseases 66

LEFT BLANK INTENTIONALLY

Introduction

THE HUMAN BEING - al-Insān - who has been created in the best possible form, is a khalīfah (vicegerent and custodian) on Earth. He needs as a prerequisite good health to fulfil his role. Traditional Islām provides guidance for all facets of human life, providing general principles in most fields including preserving health and treating disease. There are numerous verses - āyāt, in the Qu'rān which promote the health of the whole person. The Prophet Muhammad ﷺ, in his role as The Final Nabī - Messenger of Allah, lived and guided people in all aspects of life. As Ṭabīb al-Kāmil - 'The Perfect Physician', he is a model and a teacher. Early in Islamic history, the sayings and actions of the Prophet ﷺ concerning medicine were assembled into authentic collections and remained distinct. This legacy is known as the discipline of Ṭibb an-Nabawī ﷺ - the medicine of the Prophet, which illuminated and guided earlier Muslims in their development of healthcare and medicine. The Seerah and Ṭibb an-Nabawī as living traditions continue to guide us towards spiritual and physical health. Later, when Muslims came into contact with other traditions of medicine such as the Greek, Persian, Indian and Chinese traditions, they were synthesised into Traditional Medicine - Ṭibb. The 6th edition of this book includes a new section on Prophetic recipes and ingredients. I hope it will inspire you towards better health.

M. Salim Khan, 10th May 2023, Leicester, UK

1

HISTORICAL BACKGROUND

" *We have sent among you an apostle Muhammad* (صلى الله عليه وسلم) *from among yourselves, rehearsing to you our signs and instructing you in scripture and wisdom and in new knowledge.*"

(Sūrat al-Baqarah, āyah 150)

HEALTH AND MEDICINE IN PRE-ISLAMIC ARABIA

Before considering the genesis and development of Islamic medicine, it would be useful to begin by enquiring into medical conditions before Islam. Pre-Islamic Arabia provides an interesting case study for comparative analysis with later Islamic civilisation. Consideration of the ecological and socio-cultural conditions of ancient Arabia would be an appropriate starting point. The Arabian Peninsula, the Arabic term for which is Jazīrat al-'Arab, is situated on the east of the Red Sea and extends as far as the modern Persian Gulf.[1] The peninsula has considerable variations in climatic and ecological conditions which have influenced both the level and development of medicine.

Within the Arabian Peninsula, there is to be found one of the great desert regions of the world, covering an area of about 900,000 square miles. It is bordered in the west by the Red Sea, in the north by the Syrian Desert, in the south by the Arabian Sea and the Gulf of Aden and in the east and northeast by the Persian Gulf, the Gulf of Oman and the Arabian Sea.

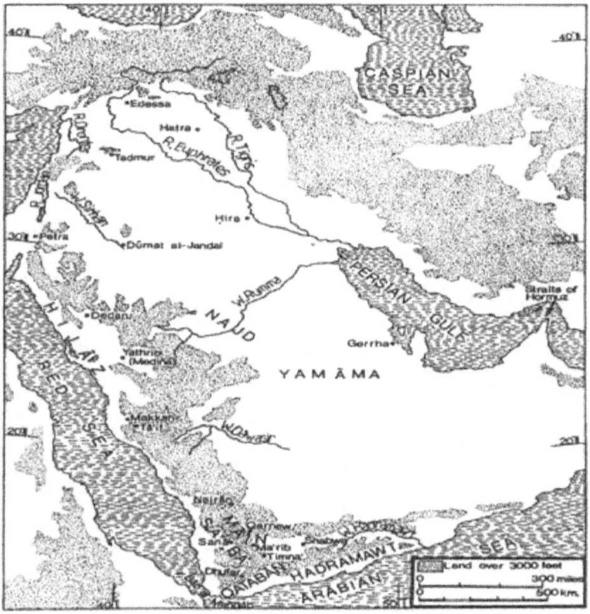

MAP 1: PRE-ISLAMIC ARABIA

There is almost always a breeze. This changes seasonally to winds of gale force, cold or hot, which chill the body, especially at night, and roast it during the summer days. The summer heat is intense, with the interior of the peninsula being dry and tolerable. Coastal regions and some highlands, however, become humid in summer, with dew and fogs at night or in the early mornings.

The winters are invigoratingly cool with the coldest weather occurring at Tā'if, with several inches of snow and ice. Summer rains in Rub' al-Khālī accompany the monsoon winds from the Indian Ocean. Dominant winds blow from the Mediterranean, swinging to the east, southeast and southwest in a great arc. Two semi-annual windy seasons occur from December to January and from May to June. These are called Shamals, which try the patience of man and beast. They are dry and transport huge loads of sand and dust, altering the shapes of sand dunes. Sharp drops in temperature are often followed by rain with wind velocities reaching gale force. On hot days the wind produces myriads of Jinn- dust devils, and the ill-famed mirage.

The vegetation throughout the peninsula is varied. Plants are primarily xerophytic – those which grow in very dry conditions. After the spring rains, long-buried seeds germinate and bloom. Date palms are grown in oases in the desert, and across the peninsula. Also found are rice, alfalfa, barley, wheat, citrus, melons, tomatoes and onions, and in the higher regions: peaches, grapes and pomegranates. Fish is in abundance in al-Ḥijāz. Ancient Arabia was well known for its production of myrrh and frankincense, two important ingredients used by the ancient civilisations of Egypt and Greece.[2]

Arabia has been inhabited by mankind since early times and consequently has had many influences from different civilisations. Most of the ancient cultures have perished, however.[3] The Arabs consider themselves to be descendants of Qaḥṭān and ʿAdnān. From these two ancestors arose numerous tribal units, forever splitting or confederating. Ancient Arabs lived as nomadic and semi-nomadic pastoralists in villages with agriculture, owning camels and sheep. Their cities had merchant and religious classes. The Quraysh of Makkah were an important group of tribes who controlled commerce and were in charge of the religious shrine known as the Ka'bah. They organised two great trading caravans which set out yearly, one in the winter, for Yemen, and the other in the summer, for Syria. These were huge convoys that brought back Oriental and African goods such as perfumes and silk. The visits of these caravans culminated in fairs with pilgrims at Makkah.

Although there existed monotheistic communities, pre-Islamic Arabia generally was polytheistic. Numerous deities were worshipped, the chiefs being al-Lāt, al- 'Uzzā and al-Manāt.[4] Promiscuity was widespread and there were mass exhibitions of nudity and rituals in which both sexes took part.[5] The status and treatment of women was inhuman. Women had no right to inheritance and were considered a commodity. If a man died, the head of the clan would throw his gown over the widow as a gesture of acquisition, which meant that the widow could not remarry anyone except the owner of the gown. If he so wished he could marry her, or keep her in a state of bondage until she died.[6] Female-child infanticide was common. Newborn girls were buried alive or thrown to their premature deaths from high places.[7] This callous and inhuman practice left deep emotional trauma on members of the unfortunate families, including the father who had to perform the brutal act.[8] Tribal chauvinism was the hallmark of ancient Arabia. Tribal wars were a common occurrence, fermented by interminable vendettas, with the killing of men and enslaving of children and women.[9] The psychological implications of living in such a society of ignorance and injustice were deep insecurity, excessive pride, guilt, and alcohol dependence. Alcohol for the pre-Islamic Arab was a psychological necessity. Life amidst oppression and stress created optimum conditions for the abuse of alcohol. It was so common that the Arabic word tājir, which means merchant, became a synonym for the salesmen of khamr - alcohol. The shops and bars of these merchants never closed during the day or night and were clearly distinguishable, being designated with special flags.[10]

It is within this ecological and socio-economic environment that the level of health and medical knowledge of the pre-Islamic Arabs needs to be located. The general level of health was poor, and harsh climatic conditions were exacerbated by social injustice, poverty and ignorance. Thus it was fertile soil for the growth and proliferation of numerous diseases. The scarcity of a clean and adequate supply of fresh water was a permanent feature. The nutritional situation was poor, with a shortage of food and a monotonous diet. There were a number of endemic diseases: leprosy, malaria, tuberculosis, rickets, scurvy numerous eye diseases and gastrointestinal diseases.[11] The pre-Islamic Arabs were familiar with the workings of major internal organs, although only in general. Surgical knowledge and practices were limited to cauterisation, branding and cupping. The care of the sick was the responsibility of the women. There is no evidence of any oral or written treatise on any aspect of medicine. There was a use of folk medicine which had interesting connections with magic. It is also interesting to note that pre-Islamic Arabia had contacts with ancient Egypt, Greece, Persia and India, where medicine was highly developed, but there is no material to suggest that it was adopted or utilised by the ancient Arabs. This is particularly surprising in view of the fact that they were well-developed in their poetry.

Medicine in the Early Period of Islam

The beginning and development of Islamic concepts and practices of health are inextricably interwoven into the general body of Islam. The organic nature of Islam encompasses the core principles of Islamic health traditions. For an understanding of the historical or conceptual aspects of Islamic medicine, a reference to Islam itself has to be made. The earlier brief sketch of pre-Islamic Arabia provides a window into the type of society in which the Prophet Muhammad ﷺ lived. The proclamation by Muhammad ﷺ, that he is the final Messenger and Prophet of Allah to mankind, began with the waḥi – Divine revelation. Until that day, Muhammad ﷺ had lived as a man amongst pagan Arabs, working as a trader. The people of Makkah, where he was born and had grown up, knew him to be a reflective, kind, and trustworthy man.

The forty years that he spent amongst them led them to regard him as al-Ameen – The Trustworthy. The foundation of Muhammad's ﷺ message was knowledge based upon higher value.

The first revelation placed knowledge as its central focus:

> "*Read! In the name of the Lord who created. Created mankind from a clot of blood. Read! Your Lord is the most bounteous who has taught the use of the pen. Has taught mankind what he did not know.*"
>
> (Sūrat al-'Alaq, āyāt 1-5)

Thus, the ignorance-based society of ancient Arabia was faced with Islam, which takes revealed knowledge as its basis. This revelation continued to be a regular feature for the next twenty-three years, and the repository of revealed knowledge became the Qu'rān which, as a source of direct and pure knowledge, addressed itself to all facets of ancient Arabian belief and conduct. Whilst on one hand, the Qu'rān stressed the oneness of Allah and His power, there was also the continued scrutiny of injustices and oppression. The Qu'rān was clear and explicit in referring to these callous practices:

> " *When if one of them receives tidings of the birth of a female his face remains darkened, and he is wrath inwardly. He hides himself from the folk because of the evil of that whereof he has had tidings, (asking himself)! Shall he keep*

the child in contempt or bury it in the dust. Verily evil is their judgement."

(Sūrat an-Naḥl, āyāt 58-59)

"*And do not marry those women whom your fathers married … it was ever lewdness and abomination, an evil way.*"

(Sūrat an-Nisā', āyāt 4-22)

Muhammad ﷺ continued his work for thirteen years in Makkah and within a decade he was able to attract most of the oppressed people, many of them slaves and poor. The small number of Muslims increasingly became victims of abuse, torture and killing. When the Quraysh saw no success in their nefarious methods, they planned to kill Muhammad ﷺ. News of this reached the Prophet ﷺ and he decided to leave Makkah and migrate to the ancient city of Yathrib. (Later, Yathrib was referred to a Madinah al-Munawwarah – the illuminated city). It was from this event that Islamic dating begins, which is known as the Hijrah. It was in Madinah that the Muslims became a community. As a community, they began to develop a tradition of health and well-being that has continued to be practised in Muslim communities throughout the world. The ecological and climatic conditions of Madinah were much more conducive to life and health than they were in Makkah. Madinah provided the conditions for the unfolding of the Sharī'ah – the Islamic way of life, of which medicine was an integral part. The Qu'rān gave general guidelines and rules on nutrition, cleanliness, marital relations, child-rearing, etc. As an example, the Qu'rān established the relationship between nutrition and behaviour. The concepts of ḥalāl – lawful and ṭayyib – wholesome, were linked to ʿamal ṣulḥah – constructive or sound behaviour; and fisq – destructive behaviour, was related to ḥarām – unlawful foods and beverages.

The Messenger ﷺ laid great stress on the importance of sound health amongst his followers. He once said:

> "*There are two gifts of which many men are cheated, health and leisure.*" [12]
>
> (Ṭibb an-Nabī- as-Suyūṭī)

Muhammad ﷺ gave specific instructions on various aspects of health-care and treated people himself. He gave detailed information on specific diseases such as leprosy and infertility, with their causes and treatments. He prohibited certain types of treatments such as cauterisation and magic, and introduced more appropriate ones. It was Muhammad ﷺ who told his companions not to embark upon treatment without adequate training. If any patient was harmed then the practitioner would have to pay diyah – compensation.[13] The Prophet Muhammad ﷺ provided the foundation for a medical tradition that considered a human being in its totality; the spiritual, the psychological and the physical within the context of a social milieu.

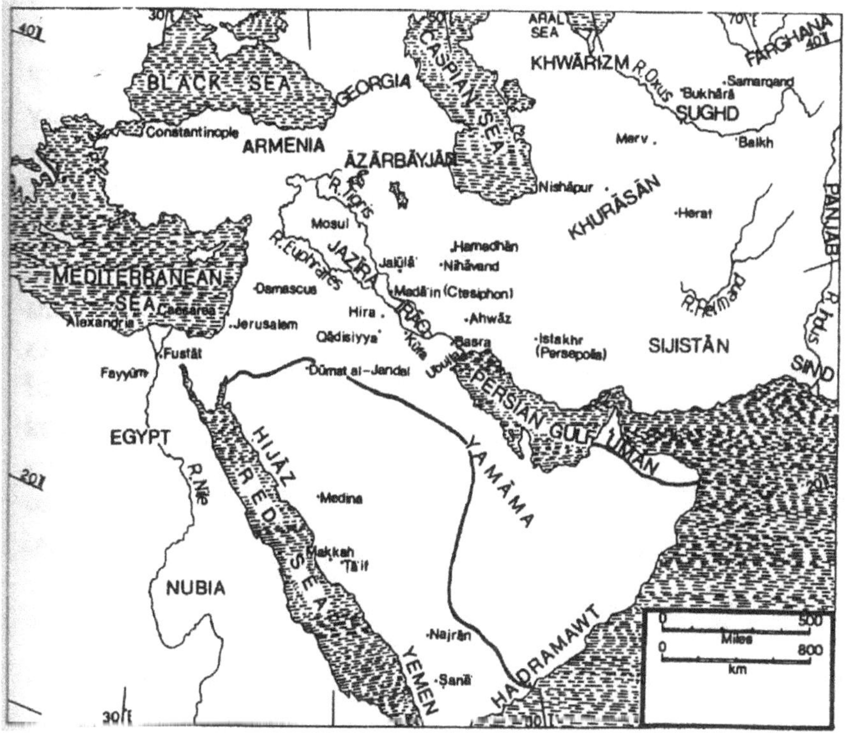

MAP 2: ARABIA AT THE TIME OF MUHAMMAD صلى الله عليه وسلم

The environment in Madinah was one where ignorance and oppression were replaced with knowledge and justice. The level of health and well-being of the people of Madinah was such that it appeared miraculous. There was an enormous difference in the level of health between the pre-Islamic eras to that in the new community of Muslims. A story from the period illustrates the health conditions:

> "One of the kings of Persia sent to Muhammad (ﷺ), a learned physician. He remained in Arabia for one or two years but no one approached him or sought his treatment. At last, he presented himself before the Prophet (ﷺ), and complained: 'I have been sent to treat your companions but during all this time no one has asked me to carry our my duties in any respect whatever' to which the Prophet (ﷺ), replied: 'It is the custom of these people not to eat until hunger overcomes them and to cease eating while there still remains a desire for food!' The physician answered: 'This is the reason for their perfect health'. He then kissed the ground in reverence and departed."[14]

The period that followed the passing away of the Prophet ﷺ is referred to as the Khilāfat ar-Rāshidah – the rightly guided rule. The Prophet ﷺ had created a generation of men and women who became the torchbearers for knowledge and justice in the traditions introduced by him, as he ﷺ put the revelation into practice. It was during this period that the famous medical centre of Jundishapur became part of the Muslim lands and continued to flourish.[15] Companions of the Messenger ﷺ, such as 'Umar and 'Alī, may Allah be pleased with them, had become masters in the matter of health and medicine. The Prophetic teachings were interpreted by these men. New cities were built according to health principles and Muslim forces and travellers were given specific instructions on the maintenance of good health. The period was an unfolding of the efforts of the Prophet ﷺ, which he had carefully implemented during his entire life. The period of the Khilāfat ar-Rāshidah was a period of rapid expansion of the Muslim community, with emphasis on collective responses to health and social care.

The Umayyad Period

In the first forty years of the Islamic calendar (661 C.E.), Mu'āwiyah of the Umayyad clan of the Quraysh tribe took over political control. The period that followed is generally referred to as the Umayyad Era. Umayyad rule lasted until 132 A.H. (750 C.E.) in the East and until 872 A.H. (1492 C.E.) in the West. It was during the Umayyad period that translations of ancient medical works began. The Umayyad prince Khālid bin Yazīd, grandson of Mu'āwiyah, was instrumental in this work. Khālid had a passion for medicine and alchemy and it was he who instructed a group of Greek Scholars in Egypt to translate the Greek-Egyptian medical literature into Arabic. These were the first translations made in Islam from one language to another; Khālid himself worked on medicine.[16] It was during this period, 120-198 A.H. (737-812 C.E.), that the most celebrated physician and alchemist, Jābir ibn Ḥayyan lived, a student of the well-known Imam, Ja'far aṣ-Ṣādiq.

Mu'āwiyah first appointed Ibn Uthal as his personal physician and this became the practice of the Umayyad governors such as Ḥajjāj ibn Yūsuf. However, it was Walīd ibn 'Abd al-Malik who, in 88

A.H. (707 C.E.), began a broad health care programme. Walīd had homes built for the blind and lepers. He developed specific treatments for the lepers and kept them separate from other patients. He also built a hospital and appointed physicians, who provided healthcare to all citizens and travellers free of charge.[17] This was the beginning of free medical care on a mass level, supported by government funds. Under the Umayyads, the Hispanic-Muslim areas of Cordoba and Granada became centres of learning. Economic prosperity and political stability along with an emphasis on knowledge and tolerance provided ideal conditions for development.

The rich and diverse flora of Spain was also a contributing factor. The development of botanical medicine was vast in Muslim Spain. Physicians like Ibn al-Bayṭār, born in Malaga in 598 A.H. (1197 C.E.) spent his early life in Andalusia, identifying and working on different plants. He also wrote a commentary on Dioscorides. His original contribution was the monumental work *al-Jāmiʿli Mufradāt al-Adwiyā wa al-Aghdhiy - The Complete [Book] in Simple Medicaments and Nutritious Items*, which dealt with some 1400 different items used in treatment. This work became an authoritative contribution to Materia Medica. Other well-known physicians were Abū Bakr ibn Samghūn of Cordoba, the philosopher and physician Ibn Bājah and Abū'l-Ḥasan al-Andalūsī who wrote extensively on plant remedies.[18]

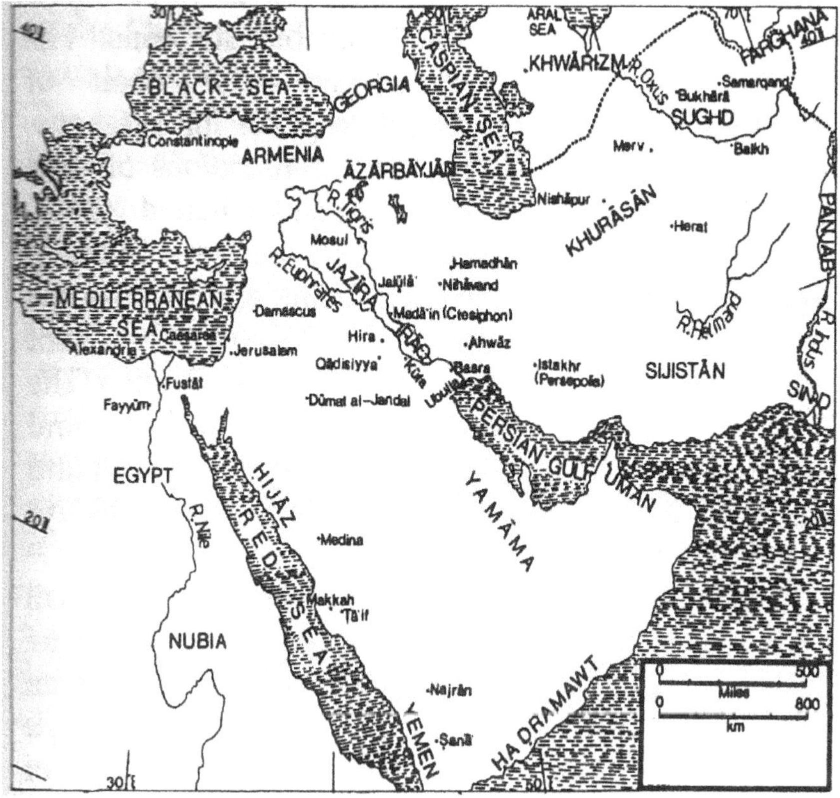

MAP 3: THE UMAYYAD PERIOD

Spain had a high level both of general medical practice and surgery. Abū'l-Qāsim az-Zahrāwī, born at Madīnat az-Zahrā', near Cordoba in 325 A.H. (936 C.E.) was one of the most capable surgeons. His systematic work, Kitāb at-Taṣrīf – *The Method of Medicine*, was the definitive guide for surgeons. The text was accompanied by illustrations of each surgical instrument and was disseminated extensively.[19] In general medicine, there were a number of scholar-practitioners in Spain writing and practising a wide range of therapies. Abū Marwān ibn Zuhr composed *Kitāb at-Taysīr fi'l-Mudāwāt Wa't-Tadbīr – The Book Facilitating the Study of Therapy and Diet*, and *Kitāb al-Aghdiyah – The Book of Diet*. Ibn Ṭufayl and Ibn Rushd were practising physicians and they also contributed to medical research and literature. The well-known Jewish philosopher and physician Abū 'Imrān Mūsā ibn Maymūn – Maimonides – who later became personal physician to Ṣalāḥuddīn, was an Andalusian and a student of Ibn Rushd and Ibn Ṭufayl. He wrote the books Kitāb al-Fuṣūl – *The Book of Aphorism*, and Kitāb Tadbīr aṣ-Ṣiḥḥah – *The Regime of Health* , as well as a number of other specific works. The development of medicine in its varied forms was helped through the particularly important contribution of Umayyad Muslim Spain. There were original contributions to surgery and internal medicine, and the creation of new disciplines and specialities such as midwifery.

The Abbasid Period

In 132 A.H. (750 C.E.) the Umayyads were overthrown by Abū'l-'Abbās 'Abdullah as-Saffāḥ who was descended from al- 'Abbās ibn 'Abd al-Muṭṭalib, a paternal uncle of the Prophet Muhammad صلى الله عليه وسلم. For the next five centuries, it was the Abbasids who dominated the socio-political life of the greater part of the Muslim world. There were major developments during the Abbasid period, particularly in medicine. The transfer of ancient medical knowledge which had begun with the Umayyads acquired new momentum during the Abbasid period. The new impetus came about for a number of reasons. The most significant event was the founding of Baghdad in 186 A.H. (754 C.E). It was Abū Ja'far, known as al-Mansūr, who founded the city of Baghdad on the banks of River Tigris in the most fertile area of Iraq. The site was also chosen for its ideal climate and absence of mosquitoes. Al-Mansūr had the city planned in such a manner as to be circular so that all the courtiers might be equidistant from the centre where the palace was built. The city was surrounded by a wall pierced by four gates. The gates were named Kufa, Basra, Khorosan and Damascus, for these were the lands and cities to which each led.

The oldest suburb and the first to rise into great importance was that known as Karkh which lay to the south-west of the original walled city and was approached through the Kufa gate. Here was built Bimāristān[20] - the hospital which became the metropolitan hospital and the cradle of the Baghdad school of medicine. Here lectured and practised all the great physicians and surgeons of Baghdad from the time of Bukt Yishu, chief physicians from Jundishapur, to the most celebrated clinician and master of Arabic medicine, Rāzī. The hospital later was referred to as 'The Old Hospital'. The situation of the hospital must have been a delightful one for in front lay the great Karkhaya Canal, a branch of the Isa Canal which joined the waters of the Euphrates to those of the Tigris.[21]

Al-Mansūr, who was the second Abbasid ruler, suffered from dyspepsia throughout his life. Having tried his personal physician, Ibn Allahaj and others in vain, he turned to physicians of the Jundishapur Medical School. Jundishapur was a flourishing centre of medical learning near the present city of Ahwaz in Iran. It was a cosmopolitan centre attracting scholars and physicians from Egypt, Syria, India, Greece and Persia. The chief physician at Jundishapur was Jurjis ibn Bukht Yishu whose reputation as a skilled clinician had reached al-Mansūr. Bukht Yishu stayed in this capacity in Baghdad until near the time of his death; when he asked al-Mansūr's permission to return to Jundishapur in A.H. 149 (C.E 769).[22]

The second phase in the development of medicine dated from the establishment of Bayt al-Ḥikmah - the Royal Library, which was based in Baghdad, the Abbasid capital. It became an important centre for the translation of medical knowledge. It was within Bayt al-Ḥikmah – literally, 'the house of wisdom' – that systemic and authentic translation as well as compilation was undertaken by competent scholars and physicians. There were separate sections dealing with literature from different languages. Jibrīl Bukht Yishu, a descendant of Bukht Yishu migrated to Baghdad from Jundishapur. He established a medical practice in Baghdad and began writing and teaching. Yuhanna ibn Masawayh, whose father worked at Jundishapur, also gained fame in Baghdad as an ophthalmologist. Ibn Masawayh became responsible for the translation of Greek texts and manuscripts into Arabic. Ḥunayn ibn Isḥāq, a student of Ibn Masawayh, was a prolific writer on medicine. He translated the work of Hippocrates, Galen and Alexandrian summaries from Greek into Arabic. His Original contribution was *Kitāb al-'Ashr Maqālāt fi'l 'Ayn – Ten Dissertations on the Eye.* Thābit ibn Qurrah compiled a work titled *The Treasury,* which became the standard text on medicine. 'Alī ibn Rabban aṭ-Ṭabarī wrote the well-known *Firdaws al Ḥikmah – The Paradise of Wisdom.* Aṭ-Ṭabarī used the medical contribution directly from Indian works. There were attractions in Abbasid Baghdad for physicians and scholars and many of them had been invited to work for their patrons. An Indian physician named Mankha was active in Baghdad translating Indian medical classics into Arabic.[23]

Within the two centuries under the Abbasids, the medical heritage of ancient civilisations became accessible to Arabic scholars. In Bayt al-Ḥikmah, scholars could work with all the necessary provisions and substantial income. The task of stocking the academy with new manuscripts became considerably facilitated due to the recent discovery of paper manufacture. Although paper was a Chinese discovery, it was introduced to the Muslim world when Samarqand was captured and the first paper manufacturing factory was established in Baghdad in 174 A.H. (794 C.E.).

The two centuries of Abbasid rule had made accessible to the Arabic-speaking physicians the greater part of the classical medical heritage. The link in this important process was the new-found city of Baghdad. The next three centuries saw the synthesis and creation of new therapies. There were a number of original thinkers and practitioners whose contribution to Islamic medicine remains alive and pulsating. Muhammad ibn Zakariyyā ar-Rāzī was born in Rey, Persia. He studied music, alchemy and later medicine. He became responsible for the main hospital in Baghdad. He was a prolific medical scholar and left many classical works such as the encyclopaedic *al-Ḥāwī – Contents on Internal Medicine.* One of the most illustrious figures of this period was Abū ʿAlī ibn Sīnā, known as 'the Prince of the Physicians'. Ibn Sīnā was born in 370 A.H. (980 C.E.) near Bukhara and travelled through Persia until his death in 428 A.H. (1037 C.E.).[24] Ibn Sīnā's most celebrated work is *al-Qānūn fi'ṭ-Ṭibb – The Canon of Medicine.* Baghdad continued to be a centre of learning with a high level of medical practice and teaching. It was during the Abbasid period that the examination and licensing of physicians and surgeons was formally organised. However, the central role of Baghdad became less important after it was devastated by Hulagu, grandson of Genghis Khan, in 640 A.H. (1240 C.E.).

Later Works

After the devastation of Baghdad, the history of Islamic medicine becomes more diverse. Fortunately, before the invasion of Baghdad, there had already been founded centres of medical learning in other parts of the Muslim world. The core concepts and practice of Islamic medicine continued to be common to various areas, although there were unique characteristics to each locality. Iran continued to be a source of medical inspiration for many years with notable physicians such as Sayyid Zayn ad-Dīn Islmā ʽīl al-Ḥusaynī al Jurjānī who wrote *Dhakhīrah Y Khwarzam – The Treasury of Medicine*, dedicated to the King of Khwarzam. In Samarqand, Abū Ḥāmid Muḥammad as-Samarqandī composed *Kitāb al-Asbāb wa'l- ʽAlāmāt – The Book of Causes and Symptoms.* The Safavid period continued with many new works on gynaecology. In Iran, European medicine was introduced through Dār al-Funūn in Tehran.[25]

In Egypt, under the Fatimids, Cairo became a centre of learning and started to attract competent physicians such as Maimonides who came over from Cordoba, Spain. Other reputable practitioners were ʽAbd al-Laṭīf al-Baghdādī, ʽAbd ar-Raḥīm ad-Dakhwar and the famous medical historian, Ibn Abī ʽUsaybiah. The physician-surgeon ʽAlā' ad-Dīn ibn Nafīs was the first to explain accurately the minor circulation of the blood. He was born in Damascus in 607 A.H. (1210 C.E.) and died in 687 A.H. (1288 C.E.).[26]

Ottoman Turkey was also an important centre of Islamic medical knowledge. The Turks built numerous hospitals which were open to all people, following the general practice in other parts of the Muslim world. The hospitals were generally regulated by trust deeds as welfare institutions. There were hospitals and medical schools built by the sultans which were both civic and military. A number of the later hospitals are still in active use in Turkey today. The language of medical instruction in Turkey was originally Arabic and was later changed to Turkish. Many of the well-known physicians wrote both in Arabic and Turkish. Initially, Turkish physicians travelled to Egypt but later Turkey became a centre for higher medical knowledge. The well-known Turkish practitioners were many including Ḥakīm Hae Pasha and Ayindoglu Umar Bey, known as 'the Ibn Sīnā of Anatolia'. It was a Turkish physician who first used smallpox vaccinations in 1059 A.H. (1679 C.E.). During Sultan Maḥmūd II's reign in 1209 A.H. (1829 C.E.) European medicine came to be taught by Dr. Bernard from Vienna, in French.[27]

The history of Islamic medicine in the Indo-Pakistan subcontinent is closely related to that of Iran. The primary language of Mogul India was Persian. Initially, the language of medicine was Persian, although later Indian scholars translated medical literature into Urdu and also developed new methods. Indian physicians began to work closely with Ayurvedic physicians which gave new impetus to Islamic medicine. India became the centre of medical learning with both traditions working very closely and at times in the same institutions and associations. India and Pakistan produced some of the most eminent physicians in later times. Akbar Arazani, author of *aṭ-Ṭibb al-Akbar – The Great Medical Work* – was one of the last physicians of the Mogul period. Ḥāfiẓ Muḥammad Ajmal Khān of Delhi, known as Masīḥ al-Mulk – 'Healer of the Nation', and one of his outstanding students Ḥakīm Muḥammad Ḥasan, known as Shifā' al-Mulk – 'Healer of the People', were the most celebrated custodians of traditional Islamic medicine in the twentieth century.[28]

2

Philosophical Conceptions of Islamic Medicine

"...This day I have perfected your way of life for you, completed my favour upon you and have chosen for you Islam as your way of life..."

(Sūrat al-Mā'idah, āyah 3)

Ilm: the Light of True Knowledge

The *Mathnāwī* by Jalāluddīn Rūmī, a classic of wisdom, contains a story called *The Disagreement about the Description and Shape of the Elephant.* The story runs as follows:

"The elephant was in a dark house. It had been brought for exhibition. Many people went into that darkness and, since seeing it [the elephant] with the eye was impossible, each person, in the dark, felt it with the palm of their hand.

The hand of one fell on the [elephant's] trunk. He said, 'this creature is like a water pipe.' The hand of another touched [the elephant's] ear. To him, it seemed to be like a fan. Another handled its leg and said, 'I found the elephant to be shaped like a pillar.' Another laid his hand on its back. He said, 'truly this elephant is like a throne'.

> In the same way, when anyone gave a description of the elephant, they understood it only according to the part that they had touched. Because of their diverse places of view, their statements differed. One man entitled it Dāl 'د', another, Alif 'ا'.
>
> If there had been a candle in each one's hand, the difference would have gone out of their words. The eye of sense perception is only like the palm of the hand: the palm has no power to reach the whole of the elephant."

The genius of Rūmī, with this story, has penetrated to the centre of the problem of knowledge. Each hand fumbles over some part of the elephant, each proclaiming what they have discovered, but none being able to relate the part to the whole. The invention of instruments that render the senses a thousand or more times acute does not reduce difficulties: if anything it increases them. Because of minute examination, one is unable to listen to what is being said at the other end of the elephant. Even if it were possible to spare the time to study different disciplines or specialities, the search for knowledge has become so intense, so much data and observations have been accumulated, that no person can ever hope to know all that others have recorded. The prospect of synthesising so much data seems an impossible task. It would seem that the very existence of an elephant has been forgotten. Consequently, the efforts are solely upon the compilation of vast catalogues of observations on the trunk, legs or tail as the case may be.

This is the unsatisfactory state in which the whole body of knowledge finds itself. It is equally true of medical science: medicine studies the human being, which is an indivisible whole of such enormous complexity that it is impossible to grasp the truth about him. Modern science, therefore, has taken him to pieces in order to study each piece separately. The modern physician, called upon to deal with a sick human being, is confronted with a truly formidable task. What renders this task so difficult is the fact that the physician is unaware of what a normal human being is, still less a sick one. He has an acquaintance with the organs of a human being and has an idea of how they work, but of the reality of the nature of the human being himself, he is woefully and confessedly ignorant. Since the renaissance in European society, the fundamental conceptions of creation, of life and of the human being, have developed in mechanistic and materialistic paths to the exclusion of any higher values. In general, this view of the world has created fundamental problems, both technological and psychological, which have placed mankind on the edge of an abyss. In this context, the ethical and holistic perspective of the Islamic tradition of health provides hopeful insights.

ISLAM: AN INTEGRATED UNITY

Any comprehensive tradition of medicine has a network of interdependent concepts and practices through which the origin, understanding, treatment and prevention of illness and maintenance of health are explained. Thus, in reality, there are close and intimately inseparable relations between the conception of a human being and health and disease.

Islam, as Dīn-I-Fiṭra – the natural way of life, has its own paradigms of knowledge. The Islamic view of reality provides a matrix in which central problems of knowledge are illuminated. Islam as a complete way of life has its own understanding of various aspects of life, including the maintenance of health and the alleviation of disease. For an understanding of the Islamic philosophy of medicine, it is necessary to have familiarity with the core values of Islam regarding the nature of creation, the position of humankind and the path of well-being.[29] Thus the health of an individual or a society can only be located within a context of Nature, society and man, as medicine is a facet of an integral view of reality. The essential outline of the philosophical tradition of Islamic healing is illuminated by the light of waḥi – Divine revelation. The cosmos is the context and the human being is the subject. This philosophical perspective considers that genuine health and happiness is the natural state of existence. However, it can only be maintained or acquired by observing the fundamental laws of creation. It is in this respect that medicine needs to be located.

TAWHID: THE FIRST PRINCIPLE AND METHODOLOGY OF UNIFICATION

Islam as a universal principle lies in the nature of creation and comprehends a human being in its totality. The whole edifice of Islam is based on an understanding of Tawḥīd – a primordial concept of the oneness and unity of all creation. The ex-nihilo created universe is perceived through this principle. Unity is a world view and a mode of comprehension, a substratum upon which Islamic sciences in general, and medicine in particular, rests. Unity as a method perceives the cosmos as a dynamic, integrated and purposeful whole. It is a method of integration and means of becoming whole and realising the profound oneness of all creation. Every aspect of Islamic thought and action rotates around the doctrine of unity, which Islam seeks to realise in a human being in his inward and outward life. Every manifestation of human existence is organically related to the Shahādah – witnessing – that there is no deity except Allah, which is the most universal way of expressing unity. From this perspective, the universe is viewed as a unity with varying levels of intelligence and will, in varying degrees. The universe is all the beings to populate the immensity of the skies, which constitutes the regions of multiplicity which extend to the spheres, the stars, the Elements, their products and humankind.

From this cosmological view, the creation is divided into two relative and continuing aspects, each influencing the other; ghā'ib – unseen or hidden, and ẓāhir – manifest. The manifest aspect of existence is accessible to sense perception and experience. These outer manifestations are āyāt – signs of the true essence. The outer and sensory manifestations are traces of a primary and unseen reality. In this paradigm of knowledge, there is an internal unity and integration between various levels of existence. Consequently, this approach, philosophically and conceptually, towards an understanding of reality has its own methodologies. One of the methods extensively employed by scholars and practitioners is the symbolic language of analogy. The classical analogy of macrocosm and microcosm suitably illustrates the point. In medical practice, the analogy of the human being with the cosmos is used:

> "The body itself is like the earth, the bones like mountains, the brain like mines, the belly like the sea, the intestines like the rivers, the nerves like the brooks, the flesh like dust and mud, the hair on the body like plants, the places where hair grows like fertile land and where there is no growth like saline soil. From its face to the feet the body is like a populated state, its back like a desolate region, its front like the east, back the west, right the south, and left the north. Its

breath is like the wind, words like thunder, sounds like thunder bolts. Its laughter like the light of noon, its tears like rain, its sadness like the darkness of night, and its sleep like death. As its awakening is like life, the days of its childhood are springing, youth like summer, maturity like autumn and old age like winter. Its motions and acts are like the motions of stars and their rotation. Its birth and presence are like the rising of stars and its death and absence like their meeting."[30]

This analogy is of profound significance and has practical implications in diagnosis and treatment. The micro-macro idea allows, through its profundity, the practitioner to penetrate beyond the physical realm. In the study of both nature and man, this idea provides the link in showing the unicity of creation, whilst demonstrating and enabling the inward relationship between them. Traditionally, the universe is the macrocosm or al-Insān al-Kabīr – 'The Great Man'. The universe is seen as one integrated body in all its spheres and gradation. It is also considered that the world has one nafs – life force, whose powers run into all the organs and cells of its body, similar to the human being. In this respect analogies from the microcosms can illustrate another difficult concept. As an example, the relationship of the universal life force of the universe, described above, becomes vivid and easy to comprehend when compared to the human life force and the human body. Conversely, analogies from the universe can be used to explain the human being by correspondence drawn from the outer aspect. This is the broad context within which an individual is located. The multifarious influences from the different levels of the cosmos are an important consideration in the ability of man towards the maintenance of equilibrium.

The Human Being: A Microcosm

The creation of the human being occupies an important place in the philosophy of Islamic medicine. The origin, nature and purpose of humankind are important guidelines for the practitioner in enabling the patient towards health and well–being. The story of human creation is vividly illustrated:

> "*Insān did We create from a quintessence (of earth); then We placed [Insān] as (a drop of) sperm in a place of rest, firmly fixed; then We made the sperm into a clot of congealed blood; then of that clot made a (foetus) lump; then made out of that lump bones and clothed the bones with flesh; then We developed out of it another creature. So blessed be Allah, the Best of creators.*"
>
> (Sūrat al-Mūminūn, āyāt 12-14)

Like all of creation, human beings are created to live and function harmoniously within themselves and their surroundings. Each person individually, and mankind collectively, are endowed with an awareness and consciousness. Creation is an amānah – trust – placed with mankind ideally and according to a design, mankind has the potential to uplift and develop himself and the rest of creation, or degrade and abase himself and his environment. Thus, each person individually and human beings collectively, are simultaneously affecting and are affected by their environment. The purpose of human beings is 'ibādah – serving and harmonising with the divine will. The outcome and result of 'ibādah is an unconditional state of sakīnah – peace and tranquillity. The concept of 'ibādah is a fundamental tenet of Islamic medical philosophy. Any evaluation of health has to take into account this central concept, as it is the key to an entire human integrity or dissipation at all levels of the being, be they psycho-physiological or psycho-spiritual. It is in this broad holistic perspective that the tradition of Islamic medicine is defined and located.

Ṭibb al-Islāmī – Islamic medicine – is the body of practices that deal with the different states of Insān – the human being in health and disease. Its purpose is to maintain health and endeavour to restore it whenever lost. Health is a dynamic state in which all functions are carried out in a ṣaḥīḥah – correct or sound, and salīmah – whole, manner.[31] This can be elaborated in that health is a dynamic condition of 'Itidāl – balance. Health is a harmonious state of forces and Elements composing the human being, as well as being external to him in conformity with the constructive principle in nature; each individual as a purposeful and integrated unity is always acting with an innate intelligence to maintain a complete and dynamic condition of balance at different levels.

The Hakim: A Symbol of Unity

The holistic perspective and unity are reflected in the discipline of Islamic medicine. Indeed the principle of unity permeates and goes deep into the very structure of the cosmos and the human self. The practitioner of this medicine is a classical example. In this figure of the Ḥakīm – sage and physician – one can see the unity of the sciences, as so many branches of a tree whose trunk is the wisdom embodied in the Ḥakīm. The Ḥakīm has always established the unity of the sciences in the minds of students by the very fact of his teaching all of the sciences as many different applications of the same fundamental principles. The Islamic teaching system as a whole and classification of the sciences, which forms the matrix are themselves dependent upon this figure of the Ḥakīm.[32]

3

The Psychological Foundations

" The question of the unity of the Divine Principle and the consequent unicity of nature is particularly important in Islam where the idea of unity (at-tawḥid) overshadows all others and remains at every level of Islamic civilisation the most basic principle upon which all else depends."

Sayyed Hossein Nasr

The Human Being: an Integrated Whole

The paradigm of Islamic psychology is essentially derived from the core of Islamic traditions, especially in the analysis of nafs – the self – and the means by which it can acquire its purpose, a state of unconditional tranquillity. Qalb – the heart, a non-material principle, is the essence of the self and has predominant control of the life of an individual. Qalb is that by which reality is perceived and interpreted. The heart, from a traditional Islamic perspective, represents the whole human being in relation to ad-dunyā – the immediate condition, and al-ākhirah – the approaching reality.[33] It is this essence which distinguishes human beings from all other created beings and constitutes the excellence which enables them to realise the truth. The heart is the point of union between jism – the body, and rūḥ – the spirit. In the Islamic order of creation, the heart is the non-material centre of the human organism, which registers and reflects conditions of consciousness. Changes can be initiated by external or internal stimuli. It is on this plane that essential functions – such as the will, thinking and synthesis – take place. Disturbance of these core functions constitutes a fundamental imbalance and disharmony within an individual. The heart is the centre of an organic whole of the psyche and soma that guides, directs and controls the human organism toward the realisation of, and unification with, the truth.

The Unity and Diversity of Nafs: the Self

The most tranquil and balanced state of the self is an-nafs al-muṭma'innah.[34] This is the ideal to which the self can aspire and as a consequence of this state, there is complete harmony within an individual in all realms of his functioning. The next state is one which is out of balance but has the ability and desire to be in tune; this condition is referred to as an-nafs al-lawwāmah, a reproachful condition in which the self is active in gaining its lost balance.[35] The unhealthiest condition of the self is an-nafs al-ammarah.[36] This is a condition of insensitivity and complete imbalance towards the destructive side of the spectrum. Thus we can see how the notion of tranquillity and balance is a central component in the evaluation of the human condition and how it has far-reaching consequences regarding the health of an individual.

The Origin and Function of Ruh: the Vital Force

Muslim physicians consider man as a psychosomatic unity endowed with a self-directing and purposeful rūḥ – vital force, which issues from the left ventricle of the heart and enables activity, growth, forms and functions appropriate to the purpose of creation.[37] The vital force is a manifestation of a combination of laṭīf – subtle particles of akhlāṭ – the Humours, and consequently, the quantity and quality of it can be modified with appropriate changes in nutrition, medication and psycho-emotional factors. The vital force diffuses itself into the remotest parts of the organism and resembles the sun in luminosity. It functions as an integrated totality in a systematic manner, according to the laws of creation. An imbalance or disharmony within the vital force is the very beginning of disease, prior to any manifestation of pathology. Thus disease *per se* begins with the vital force, whilst functional or structural changes are secondary. The nature of the vital force is dynamic and penetrating, animating every organ and particle of the human being. The existence of vital force as an integral guiding principle within the human organism, and provides the Islamic science of healing with a logical, appealing and therapeutically useful entity whilst providing a conceptual basis for the unity of disease. We can examine, in some detail, the various psycho-chemical functions of the vital force as it moves into different parts of the human organism. Although it is one pulsating eternity, in actual practice the vital force has been divided into different parts on account of its functions, making it much more valuable in diagnosis and therapy.

ASPECTS OF RUH

That part of the vital force which issues forth from the left side of the heart is referred to as rūḥ ḥaywāniyyah – the vital faculty, due to its role as a vehicle for the maintenance of life within the human being. One of the major functions of the vital faculty is that it enables organs to receive life. The expansion and contraction of the vital force are subsumed by this faculty too.

Rūḥ ṭabayyah – the natural faculty, is of two types: that which is responsible for the preservation of the individual, centred in the liver; and that which is responsible for the preservation of the species, located in the ovaries of the female, or in the testicles in the case of the male. The first type is essentially concerned with nutrition and growth while the second type is concerned with reproduction. For nutrition and growth to take place, there are a number of processes that are necessary. Attraction is the process by which food is brought into the cells and tissues and is retained by retentive force until it has been digested by a digestive faculty. When the food is suitably digested, it is assimilated and integrated into various cells and tissues.

Here, quwwah al-mughayarah – the individuation faculty, operates throughout the human body, functioning differently in the various organs according to their unique requirements. This need can be functional or structural. Each organ or organ system of the organism has an inherent natural faculty which enables it to make suitable changes in the nutrient. This process renders them one with each other in such aspects as colour and consistency. Conditions such as leucoderma, as an example, where absorption and assimilation are normal but wholeness is lacking, indicates defective individuation. Finally, the expulsive faculty is a process whereby non-nutritive matter, nutritive material in excess, and material that has served its useful purpose and is no longer required, are eliminated.

It is useful to remember that waste matter is generally expelled through natural channels of elimination. However, when such outlets are not functioning properly, waste matter is diverted to an inferior organ rather than a superior one, to a soft organ rather than a hard organ, and to a less important organ rather than a more important one. The whole strategy of the vital force indicates inherent wisdom to safeguard the core of the person from disease.

For the successful perpetuation of the species there needs to be generative and formative faculties. The generative faculty is referred to as the faculty of primary individuation and is inherent within the semen. It is the first to appear in the development of the embryo. The generative faculty deals with the formation of male and female germinal fluids which have the ability to develop various specialised cells, tissues and organs. The formative faculty gives shape, appearance and texture to the various parts, in conformity with the laws of creation.

That aspect of the vital force which is responsible for movement and sensation, and consists of cognition and conation is rūḥ nafsāniyyah – the nervous faculty, and is centred in the brain. Cognition is divided into two aspects: ẓāhir – external or conscious, and ghā'ib – the internal or unconscious. External cognition operates by means of the five senses, namely vision, hearing, smell, taste and touch. Some consider touch to be a sense that, as its sub-divisions, has pain, temperature, smoothness or roughness, softness or hardness, thus considering eight senses in total. Conation is the process by which joints and organs are moved. This results from the transmission of impulses to muscles by means of corresponding nerves. Each muscle has its own mode of movement and activity, which is initiated by thinking, which is in turn subordinate to will.

Internal cognition or perception is a complex and intricate affair which has a number of processes. The composite sense is one that is located within the interior ventricle of the brain and receives any image apprehended by the external senses and combines them into a coherent mental picture. The images formed are stored after their disappearance from consciousness and this is carried out by quwwah al-mutafakkirah – thinking, which is different from imagination. When it serves quwwah an-nāṭiqiyah – the rational mind, then it is termed thinking, whereas when it serves ilhām – intuition, then it is referred to as imagination. There is a difference between thinking and imagination. Thinking can re-arrange the impressions and can produce not only images derived from perception but can occasionally add something more which is contrary to all perception, e.g. seeing an emerald mountain. Thinking is centred within the mid-ventricle of the brain.

Intuition is the process which gives an impetus to that which has no perceptual basis and is impelling and directive in many ways. Intuition can be a source of information protecting that which it believes to be important. Intuition's function is to discover the supra-sensual ideas and it is located within the extremity of the middle ventricle of the brain. Memory is located within the posterior ventricle of the brain, together with recall. Reasoning is a component of internal cognition. These various processes originating from the external and internal sources are referred to the heart which in the light of ʿaql – an apprehending light, deals with them according to the condition of the self.

Thus we begin to see that the idea of unity permeates throughout Islamic psychology with the heart as its pivotal point.

4

Physiological Concepts

"*All the four Elements are seething in this world,*
Non is at rest, neither earth, nor fire, nor water, nor air,
Now earth takes the form of grass, on account of desire,
Now water becomes air for the sake of this affinity,
By way of unity, water becomes fire,
Fire also becomes air in this expanse because of love.
The Elements wander from place to place like pawns,
For the sake of the King's love, not, like you, for pastime."

Shams-i-Tabrīzī

The fundamental concepts in Islamic Medicine have their basis within a traditional Islamic cosmology, a matrix for all the Islamic sciences. The manifestation of existence by being is a result of the polarisation of materia prima into quwwah – energy.[38] Muslim physicians and scientists subscribe to the theory that the highest level of organisation of the cosmos is not physical but one concerned with complex energy structures. The conception of the universe in terms of energy also extends to other organisms including human beings. This approach was developed by creating a spectrum of measuring the quality of energy. The four primary qualities of heat, cold, moisture and dryness are used as a qualitative aspect of measurement, heat and cold being active and moisture and dryness passive. This concept of energy and its qualitative aspects were further developed into four basic universal symbols of the primary Elements. The macrocosm, of which the human being constitutes the microcosm, is considered the resultant of the interplay between these four primaeval Elements which are united in an unvarying pattern.

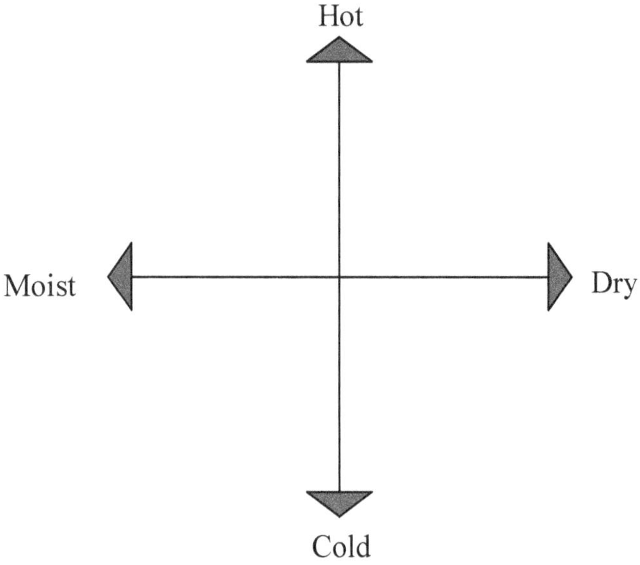

FIGURE 1: THE POLARISATION OF QUWWAH: ENERGY

ARKAN: THE ELEMENTS

The four Arkān – Elements, are a symbolic reference to actual fire, air, water and earth, and not identical *per se*.[40] The Elements are simple bodies, primary components of all minerals, plants, animals and human beings. The various orders of being depend for their existence on a particular combination of the Elements. The

Elements are subservient to the action of nature, a force present in all beings which directs and guides them.

> *"The earth is the warp and weft of the body.*
> *Heaven is man and earth women in character;*
> *Whatever heaven sends it, earth cherishes,*
> *When earth lacks heat, heaven sends heat,*
> *When it lacks moisture and dew, heaven sends them."* [39]

Earth is the Element normally situated at the centre of all existence. In its nature, it is at rest and all other Elements naturally tend towards it, however great a distance away they might be. This is because of its intrinsic weight. Earth is cold and dry. In the scheme of creation, it serves the purpose of rendering things firm, stable, lasting and heavy. It is by means of the Earth Element that other parts are fixed and held together in a compacted form. Thus it is due to Earth that the outward form is maintained. The vibration rate of Earth is slow. It is passive and receptive in nature like the female principle in creation.

Water has a position in nature which is exterior to the orbit of Earth, and interior to that of Air. This is due to its relative density. It is cold and moist. The purpose of Water in the scheme of creation lies in the fact that it lends itself to dispersion. Water provides, in the construction of things, the possibility of being moulded and shaped without permanence. Water, being moist,

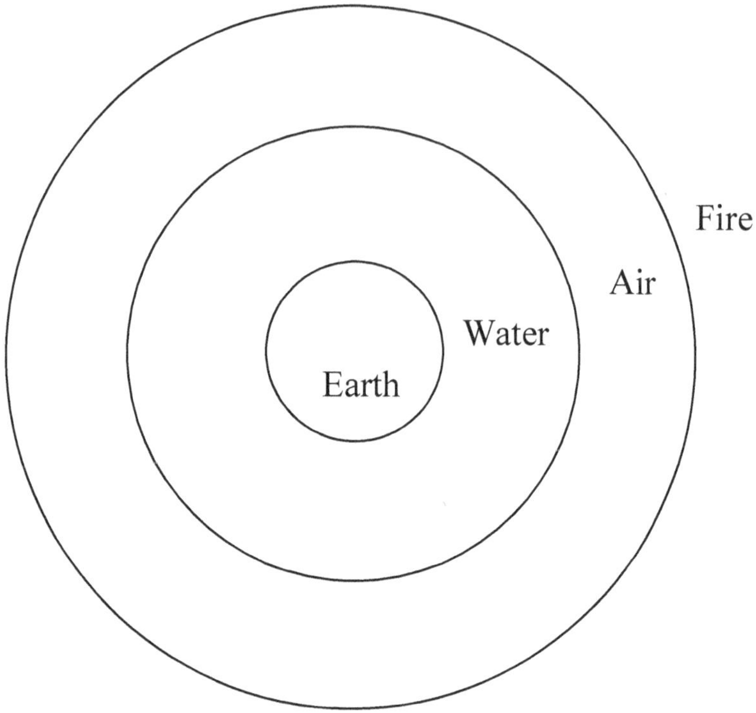

FIGURE 2: THE RELATIVE POSITIONS OF THE ELEMENTS

allows shapes to be readily fashioned. Water is a source of life as well as being essential to life.

Air occupies the position above the sphere of Water and beneath that of Fire. This is due to its relative lightness. Air is hot and moist. In nature, in the process of creation of things, its purpose is to rarefy and render things finer, lighter and more delicate.

Fire is the Element which, of the four Elements, occupies the highest position in nature. Fire is hot and dry. The part it plays in the creation of things is that it matures, refines and intermingles with all things. Its penetrative power enables it to permeate the substance of Air. It thus subdues the coldness of Earth and Water and enables their integration into various compounds. Earth and Water are required for the formation and the stability of the organs whereas the lighter Elements Air and Fire are necessary for the production and the movement of the vital forces aiding the activity of the organs.

Akhlat: the Humours

Akhlāṭ are the biological applications and extensions of the Elements. Muslim physicians conceived of the human body as a combination of al-akhlāṭ al-arbaʿah, the four primary fluids, normal and abnormal. Normal fluids are capable of being assimilated and integrated into tissue or energy, whilst abnormal fluids are unsuitable for assimilation and can be a source of imbalance and ill health. There are four primary fluids: Saudā – Black Bile, Bulghum – Phlegm, Dum – Blood and Ṣafrā – Yellow Bile. There four primary fluids in their normal state are responsible for the physiological, morphological and energy requirements of the body.

Saudā, as the Arabic word indicates, is Black Bile. It is the sediment of normal blood. Black Bile corresponds to the Element Earth, being cold and dry in nature and processing a retentive force. Its taste is midway between sweetness and astringency. Black Bile is associated with middle age and autumn and is active between 3pm to 9pm daily. Its associated organs are the spleen, the stomach and the blood. The Black Bile which enters the blood is necessary for the nutrition of organs such as the bones. Within the blood itself, Black Bile makes it thick. Black Bile which enters the spleen is used by the spleen for nutrition, to purify the rest of the body of excrementitious material, and part of it is sent to the stomach. It renders the stomach firm and active, and induces hunger by its acidity. Abnormal Black Bile can be caused by excess heat or cold, the inefficiency of the spleen, dietary indiscretions such as food containing thick and dry ingredients, and negative emotional conditions. There are several varieties of abnormal Black Bile which are a source of ill health, particularly mental-emotional diseases.

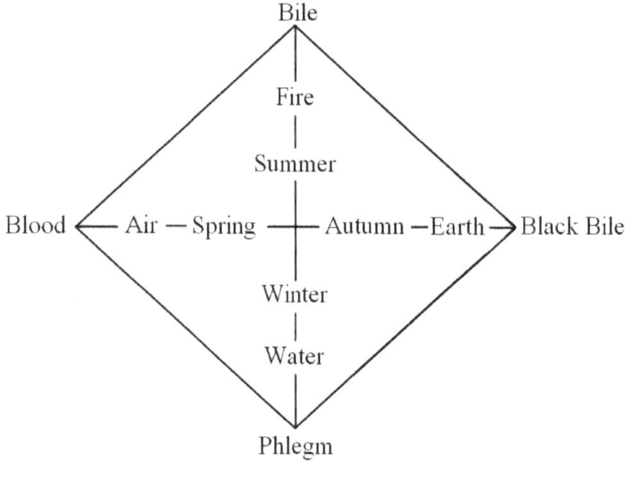

FIGURE 3: THE RELATIONSHIPS OF THE SEASONS, ELEMENTS AND HUMOURS

Normal Bulghum – Phlegm is sweet, associated with the Element Water, and is cold and moist in nature. Phlegm is dominant in old age, in winter, and during the night from 9pm to 3am. Its related organs are the kidneys, the bladder and the brain. It moves freely in the blood and joints. It possesses an expulsive force. Phlegm is unique amongst the Humours in that it can be converted into Blood when necessary. It moistens the organs and joints to prevent dryness due to excess friction and heat. There are several varieties of abnormal Phlegm and their main causal factors are lack of heat, working in water for long periods and an excess of Phlegm-producing foods such as milk and cheese.

Normal Dum – Blood is connected to the Element air, being hot and moist in nature. Its associated organs are the lungs, the blood and the liver. Blood is active in childhood, spring, and 3am to 9am. Normal Blood is red, sweet and without smell. Blood processes an attractive force. Its function is to provide nutrition to the organs and tissues. Abnormal Blood can be a result of dietary mismanagement or emotional imbalance.

Normal Ṣafrā – Yellow Bile or just Bile, corresponds to the Element Fire, being hot and dry in nature. It is active in youth, summer and 9am to 3pm during the day. Yellow Bile is light in weight, yellow in colour and possesses a digestive force. From the liver, Yellow Bile is taken into the gallbladder and the blood. The heart and the gallbladder are the associated organs. That Yellow

Bile which is taken into the blood makes the blood light and thin for easy passage through the capillaries. The Yellow Bile which enters the gallbladder serves it and activates the intestines and rectum for defecation by peristaltic movements. Abnormal Yellow Bile can be due to it mixing with other Humours, or due to a change of temperament. The causative factors can be excess heat and hot or sweet and greasy foods.

From these basic characteristics of the Humours, we can begin to understand the relationship between them, the qualities and the Elements. This simple and clear relationship begins to form a coherent picture indicating how closely and intimately interwoven relationships are between diet, seasons, health and well-being.

MIZAJ: TEMPERAMENT

Mizāj – temperament – is the dynamic state which results from the mutual interaction of primary qualities inherent within the Elements. Every being is endowed with the most appropriate temperament for the purpose and conditions of its creation. Human beings possess the most suitable temperament for the conditions of life. Temperament is the inherent tendency or predisposition to respond along particular characteristic patterns. Temperamental differences are the differences in response patterns to identical situations or stimuli. Each individual reacts according to an innate psycho-emotional pattern which makes that individual unique. The concept of temperament is a central clinical consideration, significant in diagnosis and therapy. The essential sources of determining the temperament of an individual are morphological, physiochemical and psychological signs: the practical ability to determine this and to gain an understanding of temperament must be developed over many years. Since the primary qualities of the Elements are four, the temperament of an individual is a product of the qualities of heat, cold, dryness and moisture.

Theoretically, temperament is of two kinds: balanced or imbalanced. Balanced when the opposing qualities are quantitatively equal, and imbalanced when not. Imbalances of temperament can be divided into eight varieties. In a simple imbalance of temperament, the dominance may be an excess of heat or cold without any excess of dryness or moisture, or, an excess of dryness or moisture without any excess of heat or cold. However, simple imbalances do not last for long as they soon become compound. For example, an imbalance in the direction of excessive heat will promptly lead to dryness.

Compound temperaments are those that have two dominant qualities, such as hot and moist, hot and dry, cold and moist, or cold and dry. There is no coupling of heat with cold or dryness with moisture. The aforementioned eight imbalances, four simple and four compound, have further gradations of each type into a further four degrees, depending on the degree of the imbalance. Thus, in practice, there can be multi-level gradation depending on the condition of imbalance. Imbalances can be of two kinds. The first kind is *with morbid matter*, where temperament has become imbalanced due to an introduction of matter in the body, such as Phlegm or Yellow Bile. The second kind is *without morbid matter*, which can arise per se and not from any morbid matter, e.g. cold when exposed to snow.

There are other variations, such as females are generally colder in temperament than males. They have a smaller build and have more relaxed tissues and muscles. Traditionally, the human lifespan on earth is divided into four broad periods: growth, which extends to twenty-eight years; maturity, which lasts up to forty years; middle age, which extends up to sixty years; and finally, senility. The period of growth is balanced regarding heat but has an excess of moisture. During maturity, there is a moderate excess of heat whilst in middle-age and old age there is an increasing proportion of cold.

Temperaments of the Organs

As mentioned earlier, each being as a whole is endowed with the most suitable temperament for itself and likewise its individual parts and organs. In the case of human beings, each organ has also received the appropriate temperament requisite for its function, nature and conditions. There are some which are hot, others cold, and others dry or moist. The degrees of dryness are as follows: hair is the driest of the tissues as it is formed of smoky vapours solidified by the evaporations of moisture. The darker the hair, the dryer it is. Next are the bones, which are the hardest organs. They are slightly moister than hair as they are formed of blood with much Black Bile and absorb moisture from the muscles attached to them. This is the reason that a number of animals derive nutrition from them, whereas this is not the case with hair. Following in descending order of dryness are: cartilage, ligaments, tendons, membranes, arteries, veins, motor nerves, the heart, sensory nerves and skin. The coldest component of the body is the Phlegm, followed by in descending order of coldness: hair, bones, cartilage, ligaments, tendons, membranes, nerves, the spinal cord, breast, testicles, lungs, liver, spleen, kidneys, muscles and skin. The hottest organ in the body is the vital force and the heart, followed by: blood, liver, muscles, spleen, kidneys, artery walls and skin. As a general principle, the organs rich in Blood are hot and those poor in Blood are cold in temperament. As it is obvious from the above gradations, the skin is the most balanced organ, and in particular the skin of the tips of the fingers.

Temperaments of Medicines

> "*Lo! The righteous shall drink of a cup whereof the mizāj (Temperament) is of camphor.*"
>
> (Sūrat al-Insān, āyah 5)

In traditional Islamic medicine, all living objects are categorised according to temperament based on the primary qualities of heat, cold, dryness or moisture. The temperament of articles of diet, items of aesthetic value, e.g. gemstones, and medicines, are generally tested on healthy human beings. These tests have rigorous standards upon which Materia Medica is built. There is a system of gradation based on the degree of change that a given substance can induce within a balanced individual. There are in fact an infinite number of gradations manifested in the equally infinite number of differences between substances, as was the case with temperament within individual persons. Thus, each substance has its unique temperament, modified by climate, habitat, etc. Compound medicines also have their own temperament which in practice becomes much more difficult to access. Thus, in actual therapy, the physician needs to be conversant with the temperament of the articles of diet and medicine. In practice, it takes many years to acquire and develop the practical art of analysis and diagnosis. We can begin to see the central importance of the evaluation of temperament in diagnosis and therapy. Specific details of signs of temperament will be discussed in a later chapter on diagnosis.

Aʿda: The Organs

The structure and functions of the human body form an extensive field of study requiring years of dedicated work. In this sub-section, we wish to indicate an Islamic approach to the study of anatomy and physiology, rather than to supply extensive details. The unitary nature of knowledge in the Islamic sciences can be appreciated when studying human anatomy and physiology. According to the Islamic science of medicine, every cell, tissue and organ is created in a most perfect structure to fulfil its functions. The organs are primarily formed from the co-mingling of the fluids just as the fluids are derived from the primary Elements. Every organ is endowed with an innate force for nutrition by which it absorbs, retains, assimilates and integrates its own nutrition and excretes the toxic and waste matter harmful to life and health. The constituents of the human body can be divided into simple and compound organs. The aʿḍā mufridah – simple organs are those parts in which the visible and perceptible constituents convey the same name and definition as the whole. They are the bones, cartilage, nerves, tendons, ligaments, arteries and joints, membranes and flesh. These constituents are said to be homogeneous, as their particles or cells are of similar types.[41]

Aʿḍā' murakkabah – compound organs, are the organs of which the comprising parts, irrespective of size, differ in nature as well as name from the whole organ, e.g. hand. Thus, a part of the hand cannot be called a hand. Compound organs are divided into a hierarchy of importance. The vital or principal organs are the heart, the brain, the liver and the generative organs. These are the centres of various functions and activities, absolutely necessary for the life of an individual and the species. The rest of the organs are auxiliary to the vital organs or are those which are instruments of their functions. The lungs are an example of the latter type.

The following table indicates the groups of organs as well as how they relate to each other:

Vital Organs	Preparative Organs	Auxiliary Organs
Heart	Lungs	Arteries
Brain	Stomach and Liver	Nerves
Liver	Stomach	Veins
Testis/Ovaries	Generative Organs	Penis, Ducts, Uterus etc.

We can begin to appreciate the unitary nature of anatomy and physiology with its gradation. Information and an understanding formulated in such a manner and methodology can be helpful to the physician in immediately evaluating the seriousness of any conditions upon taking up the case.

Data organised in this systemic manner, based on natural laws can be of much more value in the analysis of a given individual's health status than information derived from artificial classification which ignores the order of creation.

In this chapter, a brief outline of the main physiological concepts used in traditional Islamic medicine has been described. The nature of the traditional healthcare approach in Islam is holistic and subtle, leading to a logical unity between structure and function.

5

LIFE BALANCE

"He erected heaven and established the balance, so that you would not transgress the balance. Give just weight – do not skimp in the balance."

(Sūrat ar-Raḥmān, āyāt 5-7)

Health is a dynamic condition of balance that is the result of an individual's ability to cope with internal and external influences. The individual needs not only to create an internal balance within him but to adapt to social, ecological and spiritual conditions.[42]

The Ḥakīms over many centuries have delineated essential factors that are fundamental to the maintenance of life and health. They are referred to as the 'six essential factors' and any imbalance in them ultimately results in disease and premature death.[43]

The 'six essential factors' are as follows:

- Ecological conditions
- Mental and emotional aspects
- Sleep and wakefulness
- Diet and nutrition
- Physiological movement and rest
- Retention and elimination.

Ecological Considerations

The multiplicity of influences of the universe upon any individual is numerous, from the most subtle, such as the spirit, to the most gross, such as the sun. Air is necessary for the maintenance of life and health and is an elementary constituent of human beings. Man remains healthy as long as the air is balanced and free from pollution. Balanced air is free from fumes, chemicals, smoke and excess water vapour. Good quality air is that which is pure, clean, and free from the vapours of ditches, ponds, waterlogged fields and foul gases from animal or vegetable remains. Good quality air is air which is open to fresh breezes, especially air that comes from plains and high mountains. There are two essential functions of air: the first is conditioning, and the second is the purification of vital force.

Conditioning refers to the moderation of the temperament of the vital force. The vital force is moderated by air inhaled through the lungs and taken through the pores adjoining the arteries. The air that surrounds our bodies is generally much cooler than the normal temperature of the vital force. The contact and admixture of the vital force with balanced air prevents the vital force from becoming abnormal. Purification is the process whereby toxic vapours and substances are eliminated during expiration. The vital force is moderated by getting cooled during inspiration and purified during expiration.

Air has different effects depending upon its qualitative nature. Hot air is relaxing and produces dispersion. Moderate heat makes the complexion red, drawing blood toward the surface. Excessively hot air can turn the complexion yellow and disperses blood, producing excessive sweating and reducing the quantity of urine. It impairs digestion and causes excessive thirst. Cold air makes the body firm, strengthens digestion and increases the quantity of urine. Cold air hinders elimination and prolongs stagnation. It separates water and diverts it toward the kidneys, leading to solid stools. Dry air makes the body thin and the skin dry and rough. Moist air softens the complexion and increased moisture.

Air is subject to changes which have health implications. These changes can be normal or abnormal. Seasonal variations are normal changes. Spring is considered the best season. Its temperament is suitable for the growth and preservation of life in general, and the blood and life force in particular. It is the time when the trees sprout. Spring, out of all the seasons, is the most balanced and tends to promote natural moisture and subtle heat. It promotes a rosy complexion and activates the Humours but does not disperse them as in summer. Spring is a particularly suitable season for children and those in the stage of puberty. During spring the activation of the Humours leads to certain diseases, particularly chronic diseases. Diseases of spring are nose bleeding, rupture of blood vessels, and skin conditions such as abscesses. Individuals with a phlegmatic temperament may suffer from diseases such as apoplexy and paralysis.

Summer tends to disperse the Humours and the vital force, causing enfeeblement of bodily functions. During summer there is a decrease in the quantity of Blood and Phlegm with consequent changes to the quality of the Humours in general. Yellow Bile is increased during this season, giving a yellow tint to the complexion. During the latter part of summer, there is a greater accumulation of Black Bile due to the dispersion of the lighter Humours. Diseases of summer tend to be of short duration as the heat tends to mature and eliminate any diseased matter. However, in individuals of low vitality, excess heat may cause debility. Diseases of summer tend to be due to the migration of the Humours from the upper parts to the lower, such as diarrhoea. Febrile conditions are also common, as well as gangrene, and infections of the eyes and ears

Of all the seasons, autumn is the one when diseases are most prevalent. The reason for this is that during autumn there is less Blood as it is dissipated by the other Humours, leaving excessive Black Bile. As this period starts to become cold there is a reduction of elimination and purification thus diverting Humours inwards. Diseases of autumn are due to an excess of Black Bile such as melancholia, cancer and joint pains. The expulsive faculty is weakened during autumn.

Winter aids digestion. Individuals who tend to have a sedentary lifestyle, with excessive food intake during winter, are predisposed to depressive conditions. It is a period which is cold and useful for reducing Yellow Bile. Winter diseases are usually phlegmatic. The common cold and its effects are prevalent at this time of the year. Winters which are particularly long and harsh are unfavourable to the old. There are also increased attacks of nervous disorders during this season.

Appropriate measures relevant to each season will be discussed in the chapter on treatment.

Mental and Emotional Factors

The core of an individual is the spirit which manifests itself through the mental and emotional channels. The different shades of emotions can be either, positive, creative and life-enhancing or negative, destructive and death-promoting. Each emotion, depending on its quality and severity, influences an individual and in particular their vital force. In general, the movement of the vital force is outward and gradual in beneficial states, such as happiness or pleasure, whereas in conditions of sorrow, depression or fear the movement of the vital force is inward. Coma, or at times death, can occur due to sudden inward movement of vital force, as in shock. Any prolonged movement toward negative aspects can predispose an individual towards serious mental-emotional and physical illness.

Sleep and Wakefulness

Sleep is an important factor in the preservation and promotion of health. The quantity and quality of sleep is a significant cause of disease. Sleep removes fatigue and regulates the flow of excretions due to the activities of the day. During sleep, the innate heat is directed inwards, helping to promote digestion, growth and healing. It is due to the inward movement of the innate heat that the exterior of the sleeper becomes cold. The most beneficial sleep is night-sleep, undisturbed, after a light nutritious meal. Excess sleep can dispose one towards nervous diseases and dull intellectual functions, and cause an accumulation of excess cold Humours. Shortage of sleep is predisposed to create excess dryness with diseases such as mental confusion, itching and irritability. The effects of wakefulness are opposite to that of sleep.

Diet and Nutrition

Amongst the various causes responsible for health and disease, are articles of food and drink. Each separate item of food and drink individually, as well as in their different combination, have a specific effect on human health. The following factors also need to be considered: the manner of eating, the psychological state of the person, the time of day and year, and the quantities and qualities of the foods and drinks. In the Qu'rān foods and drinks are divided into two broad categories: Ḥalāl – lawful, and Ḥarām – unlawful. The first category is further divided into a range of foods and drinks which are particularly health-promoting and are referred to as ṭayyib – wholesome. Each item of nutrition is further studied as to its qualitative aspect of being hot, cold, dry or moist. These four primary qualities are then related to one of the four primary Humours. The quality and quantity of food and drinks is an essential tool in the maintenance and restoration of health. If we take water as an example, as an Element it is present in food and drinks, enabling food towards liquefaction, transportation and absorption. There are several types of water and that which is conducive to health should have the following qualities:

- It should be light in weight;
- Have a pleasant taste;
- Be easily turned hot or cold;
- Enabled for quick and easy cooking;
- Have no odour or colour;
- Should quench the thirst.

An example of water with these qualities is the water from the Zamzam spring in the valley of the Ḥijāz in Makkah.[44] The best type of water is obtained from springs where the ground is pure and free from abnormal conditions, preferably from rocky mountains which are exposed to sun and fresh air. Rainwater and water collected after a storm, in an area free from pollution, is also health-promoting. However, rainwater has a tendency to set up putrefactive changes, due to its lightness. Water from snow or hail is generally impure as a drink. In hot climates or summer, ice and iced water may be used in moderation provided it is made from a pure water supply. Individuals suffering from conditions such as neuralgia or gastrointestinal inflammation should refrain from iced drinks. Well water may be used, although it should be frequently lifted from the well. Water from marshes should be avoided, as well as water containing heavy metals such as lead. Water infested with such things as leeches, frogs, etc. should not be used. Water rich in specific trace elements such as zinc or sulphur can be helpful in specific disease conditions.

Physiological Movement and Rest

Any form of activity, whether it is prolonged or short, mild or vigorous, produces heat in different degrees. However, prolonged mild activity produces a greater dispersion of Humours. Different occupations produce their impact on health and cause specific diseases. An occupation such as that of a washer man or woman, undertaken over a long period, will result in a cold and moist condition. Likewise, a blacksmith can be disposed towards excess heat and dryness because of the nature of his work. Rest is cooling and moistening, since during rest there is little or no excitation of heat, and little or no inward accumulation of matter which subdues the heat.

Retention and Elimination

Any imbalance in retention and elimination can be a cause towards disease. For the maintenance of health, there needs to be a balance between proper retention and elimination.[45] An imbalance in retention can occur when the expulsive force is weak or the retentive force is excessively strong. Improper digestion can lead to prolonged obstruction of eliminative channels due to thick and viscid matter. Diseases of excessive retention are also moist and complex. Elimination or loss of matter occurs when conditions are contrary to those of retention. The diseases that occur due to excess elimination are cold and debilitating.

6

Diagnosis

"*The physician should be of tender disposition, of wise and gentle nature, and more especially an acute observer, capable of benefiting everyone by accurate diagnoses; that is to say, by rapid deduction of the unknown from the known; and no physician can be of tender disposition if he fails to recognise the nobility of the human being; nor of philosophical nature unless he knows logic, nor an acute observer unless he be strengthened by God's guidance.*"

Chahar Maqala of Samarqand

Indications of Health

Before considering disease and its symptoms it is important to have an understanding of health. The signs of a healthy person with a balanced temperament are as follows:

- The complexion of an individual is pleasing, with shades and colours that are normal to their biological environment;
- Body build is medium, neither too lean nor too heavy;
- Hair is not too profuse nor scanty;
- The feel of the body is balanced in respect of heat, cold, moisture and dryness;
- Sleep and wakefulness are moderate;
- Movements are free and easy;
- Intellectual functions and memory are good;

- Habits and behaviour are balanced between timidity and assertiveness, anger and calm, leniency and Humour, pride and humility;
- Growth and repair are rapid whereas deterioration is slow;
- Dreams are interesting and pleasing.

The healthy person enjoys food, digests and assimilates normally, and their excretory functions are regular.[46]

Classifications of Disease

It has been emphasised that Ṭibb has an integrated approach towards health and disease in the context of the spiritual, ecological and social environment. Over centuries, the practitioners of Ṭibb have evolved several classifications of disease. A disease is an imbalance that disturbs the harmony and balance which is natural to human beings. A disease may be described as medical, surgical, chronic or acute depending upon its nature or treatment. However, in any disease condition, the unity of the person must not be forgotten, even though at any given moment the disturbance may be centred on a specific level or organ. There is a hierarchical division of disease from above downward and from within outward, the most important being above and within. This gradation can be depicted in diagrammatic form, the most central and crucial being the spiritual level and the least important being the peripheral.

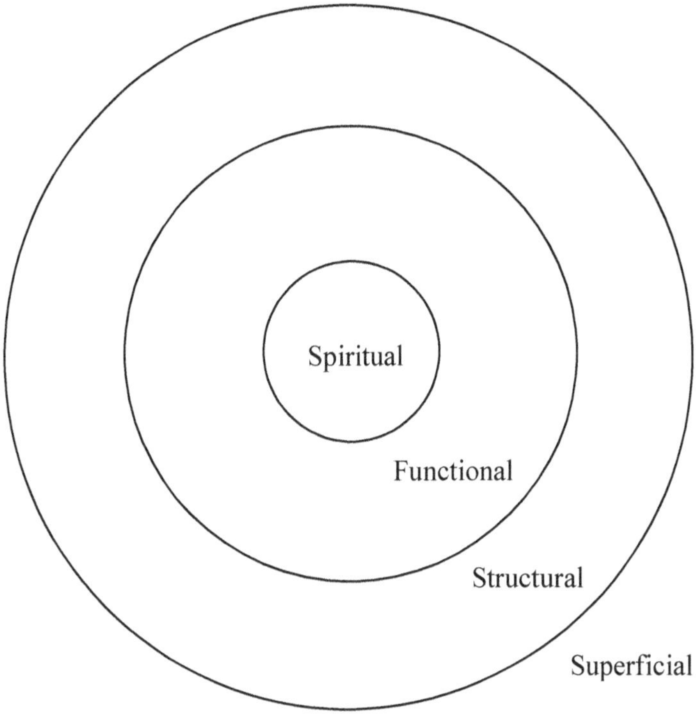

FIGURE 4: HIERARCHICAL CLASSIFICATION OF DISEASES

The most important and highest level of an individual is the spiritual level. Disturbances on this level constitute the most fundamental imbalance. Imbalances on the spiritual level manifest in the disturbance of consciousness and mental functions. Conditions such as suicide, schizophrenia, delirium and total insanity are the result of disturbances on this plane.

Functional diseases are disturbances that are manifested in imbalances of temperament. These imbalances may be simple dominance of the active qualities of heat or cold or the passive qualities of dryness or moisture. However, simple imbalances are soon changed into compound imbalances – a dominance of two qualities – such as: hot and moist, hot and dry, cold and moist, or cold and dry. These imbalances of simple or compound type can arise either with morbid matter or without morbid matter.

Structural diseases are diseases of the structure which may be of simple organs such as the bone, or of compound organs like the stomach. Structural diseases may affect the size, number or form of an organ. Superficial diseases are diseases that manifest themselves on the skin, hair or other areas of the complexion. Within the hierarchy, this is the outermost aspect of an individual. However, superficial diseases are a reflection of the inner workings of the individual.

Signs of Temperaments

The concept of temperament is of great importance in clinical practice, particularly in diagnosis. The notion of temperament is broad enough to encompass both the structural and the functional aspects of an individual.[47] The signs and indications of diagnosing a temperament are many. Here we will consider the major ones.

Body build is a helpful indicator of evaluating the temperament of a person. A muscular body that is well-developed is a sign of heat and moisture, particularly when it is firm and solid. Poor muscular development with a deficiency of fat is an indication of dryness. A fat, flabby and cold body is a reflection of a cold temperament.

Complexion is also a sign which helps in the understanding of temperament. A pale or bluish tinge is cold and shows a lack of Blood. Yellow complexion points to an excess of heat and Yellow Bile. A dark complexion illustrates heat and dryness, whereas red or rosy colour shows heat and moisture.

As well as these general signs, there are more specific indications that help in diagnosing an individual's temperament:

People of hot temperament have a broad chest, a well-developed body with good muscular growth, especially around the joints. This is due to the fact that heat promotes growth. These people are likely to have dark hair which is thick, profuse and which grows rapidly. Their completion may be dark or rosy. Their body is likely to feel hotter than that of a balanced person. The discharges or excretions of a person with a hot temperament are likely to have strong odours, high colour and full maturity. For individuals whose temperament is abnormally hot, there may be additional signs and symptoms: they may feel uncomfortable in the heat, have excessive thirst, irritation and burning in the pit of the stomach, bitter taste in the mouth, intolerance of hot foods and drinks, craving of cold foods and drinks, and excessive anger. All of these symptoms could get worse in summer and around midday.

Persons of cold temperament have the opposite signs and symptoms to those of hot-tempered individuals. Cold hinders growth and maturity and these individuals are likely to have fat bodies that feel soft, flabby and cold to the touch. They are also likely to have thin, scanty hair which is slow to grow. Their complexion is more inclined towards pale or white and chalky. Their excretions or discharges such as urine and perspiration are inconsistent, sluggish and without strong odour. They are more likely to be sluggish and sleep excessively. In individuals whose temperament is abnormally cold, there will be additional signs of weak digestion, absence of thirst, dislike of cold drinks and foods, craving of hot drinks and foods, cold and catarrhal discharges, laxity of joints, and their symptoms becoming worse during winter and at night.

People of moist temperament are more likely to have similar symptoms to those of cold temperaments. However, in abnormally moist individuals there will be additional signs of excessive salivation, nasal discharges, diarrhoea, excessive sleep, puffiness of the body, especially under the lower eyelids, and intolerance of moist foods and habitat.

Persons of dry temperament have dryness and roughness of the skin, a thin body, with prominent joints and rapid growth of hair. In cases of abnormal dryness, there may be additional indications such as insomnia, wasting, intolerance of dry foods, craving for moist foods and drinks, rapid absorption of light oils and worsening of symptoms in autumn.

PULSE

In the repository of wisdom and skills of Islamic medicine, one of the subtle and important tools for evaluation of health and disease is the pulse.[48] The pulse is the movement and contraction of the heart. The purpose of this movement is to condition the vital force. Each pulse beat consists of two movements and two pauses. Thus there is expansion, followed by a pause, then contraction, accompanied by a pause. Traditionally the pulse is felt by palpating the radial artery at the wrist. The reason for feeling the pulse at this point is that it is accessible and can be examined without embarrassment to the patient, and it is in direct continuity with the heart. It is important that when the patient is examined, the stomach should not be full and the patient should be at ease. The person examining the pulse needs to be calm and in a balanced state of health. The necessary sensitivity and practical skill in examining the person has to be developed under supervision. The study of the pulse is complex and can be approached from different perspectives. However, here it is only possible to discuss the general principles governing the study of the pulse. The physicians have laid down a number of features of the pulse that provide valuable information helpful in the evaluation of health and the diagnosis of disease:

Size: the size of the pulse is noted by examining the degree of its expansion regarding the height, length and breadth. Thus in terms of size, the pulse has nine varieties. These are: long, short or medium in length; broad, narrow or medium in breadth; and low, high or medium in depth. A pulse is considered long if it is longer than the pulse of the hypothetical absolute balance. A long pulse is an indication of excess heat and excess activity. A short pulse is the opposite of the long one, indicating low heat and low activity. A medium-length pulse indicates a balanced individual. The width – or breadth – of the pulse gives an estimate of the amount of moisture. A wide pulse indicates excess moisture, whereas a narrow pulse is the opposite, with medium-breadth being the balanced state. The depth of the pulse is used to elicit the level of activity. A raised pulse points to a high level of activity, with its opposite pointing to a contrary state. A medium-depth pulse indicates a balanced level of activity.

Temperature: the temperature of the pulse indicates the quality of the Humours. A hot pulse indicates excess heat, whereas a cold pulse points to a lack of heat. A moderate pulse indicates balance.

Duration of pulse: pulse is rapid or hurried when the period between two beats is less than normal. A rapid pulse is indicative of a fading vital force. The pulse is slow when this period is long, and this shows strong vital force. A medium pulse is between these two extremes.

Constancy: a pulse may continue to be constant, or vary, in respect of the feature illustrated above. A constant pulse is an indication of good health, whereas an irregular pulse points to weakness or disturbance. Irregular pulse can have numerous permutations too detailed to be mentioned in this work.

Strength or quality of impact: strength of the pulse gives an indication of the quality of the vital force. The pulse which is felt by the pores of the fingers can be strong, which during expansion strikes forcibly against the practitioner's fingers. This variety of a strong pulse indicates a strong vital force. A weak or feeble pulse, the opposite of the strong type, is a pointer toward slow vitality. A medium pulse is midway between the two types.

Speed or duration of cycle: speed of the pulse is an indication of a person's need for oxygen. The speed of the cycle of the pulse may be quick in which the duration of individual beats is shorter. This pulse is an indication of an individual's need for a greater amount of air. A medium type is between the two types, reflecting a balanced condition.

Consistency or elasticity: the elasticity of the pulse may be hard, pointing to excess dryness or soft and easily compressible, reflecting excess moisture. A pulse of medium consistency is indicative of balanced moisture.

URINE

The excretion and discharges from specific organs and the general body provide diagnostic indications. Urine as an example provides information about the functional states of the kidneys, digestive system, liver and spleen. However, it is important to consider the following conditions:

- Urine should be collected in the morning before any drinks or foods have been eaten;
- No substance which can alter the colour of urine should be taken, such as saffron;
- The person giving the sample of urine should not be unduly tired or mentally excited.[49]

Important points to be considered in using urine in diagnosis are colour, density, turbidity, sediment, quantity, froth and odour.
Normal urine of a healthy adult is of moderate density and pale yellow in colour. It is free from an unpleasant smell, although it is not odourless. The sediments are not abnormal and there should be no irritation or burning.

The yellow colour has many shades such as orange, saffron, etc., and these different shades are an indication of over-activity and heat. Any shade of green points to a cold temperament, as does white. Dark colouring points to an excess of Black Bile and excessive combustion of Humours.

The density of urine can be thin, medium or thick, each significant. Thick urine is a sign of defective maturation or elimination. Thick but clear urine is an indication of Phlegm. Thin urine is due to incomplete maturation or weakness of kidneys, and obstruction or intake of fluids. Turbidity of urine is due to an admixture of rīḥ – gaseous air – with heavy particles. If urine is at first clear but becomes turbid on standing it indicates that the body is trying to mature the morbid matter. Turbid urine which clears upon standing but leaves a deposit of coarse particles indicates successful maturation. Turbidity of urine can also be due to the elimination of matter from the liver, spleen or kidneys. In such cases, the findings need to be correlated with the other diagnostic methods of pulse and stool.

Odour from a diseased person's urine is different from that of a healthy individual. Odourless urine is a sign of a cold temperament and immature Humours. Foul-smelling urine can be a sign of ulceration in the kidneys or urinary tract. Sweet-smelling urine indicates a dominance of Blood, whereas pungent smells point to an excess of Yellow Bile. An acidic or sour smell shows increased Black Bile.

The different types and amounts of sediment also provide diagnostic information. Any sample will have normal and abnormal sediments. The quantity and quality of sediment are in chemical and physical aspects. In spite of adequate fluid intake, scanty urine passed with ease is a sign of low vitality and recovery.

Stool

Occasionally conclusions may be derived from the condition of the stool of a person. Normal stools are compact, well-formed and passed at regular periods; without griping or irritation. The stool should usually be almost odourless, free from froth, and faintly yellow in colour.[50] In any consideration of stool analysis, the important factors are quantity, consistency, colour and sediment which may have been eliminated from the system through the stools. Quantity may be judged by taking into account the amount of food consumed. Large stools are indicative of a dominance of Humours, whereas scanty stools indicate a deficiency. The liquid stools point to indigestion, weakness of mesenteric vessels or possible obstruction. Stools with froth, instead of being firm and compact, point to rīḥ or excess of heat. Dry stools point to cold, polyuria or intake of dry foods.

Excess change in stool colour may be indicative of a disease process. Hyperfunction of Yellow Bile can change the colour of the stools to excess yellow, whereas pale stool indicates a lack of maturation. White stools can point to a lack of or obstruction of bile ducts.

Black stool may point to an excess of Yellow Bile, which may be indicative of serious illness. Pus and blood may also be a sign of serious illness. It is important to eliminate extraneous factors such as specific foods and medication which may alter the various colours or consistency of stool.

7

Preventative Aspects

"Children of Adam! Wear fine clothing in every mosque and eat and drink but do not be profligate. He does not love the profligate."

(Sūrat al-Aʿrāf, āyah 29)

Personal Hygiene

One of the principal objects of the Islamic healthcare tradition is to prevent suffering and disease prior to any clinical manifestation. A person's entire life is guided and directed towards wholesomeness and longevity with the main emphasis on prevention. Islam as an ethical and holistic way of life deals with the spiritual and physical aspects of an individual and the community. On the spiritual and ethical levels, teaching and practice harmonise the inner consciousness with the outer reality of creation. The clear and sublime perspective focuses and liberates the individual from doubt, confusion and subjugation to others and positively helps to give purpose and meaning to life. This wisdom is interwoven into daily living. A description of the daily routine will give an insight into the preventative dimension.

An individual is expected to get up early in the morning at fajr – dawn – before sunrise. After defecation and urination, the person cleans both his hands with clean water and properly washes the anus and genital areas. This is called istinjā'.

The person then begins the process of wuḍū'. First, the hands are washed up to and including the wrists. This is followed by cleansing of the mouth, including teeth and gums. The teeth are cleaned with miswāk – a traditional plant used from the early Islamic period for cleaning teeth and oral hygiene.[51] The miswāk cleanses the teeth and contains antibacterial substances that destroy the harmful germs in the mouth which cause infection and tooth decay. These wooden sticks are ecological and natural as well as safe and economical. The mouth is washed three times with clean water. Next, both nostrils are cleaned internally of mucus and externally of dust. The nose is washed with clean water using the left hand. Next, the whole face is washed beginning from the hairline all the way down to the chin, and from one earlobe to the opposite earlobe. The cleansing of the face is followed by washing both arms from the wrists, up to and including the elbows. After this, moist hands are passed over the head. The tips of the fingers are used to clean the ears. Finally, this is completed by washing both feet up to and including the ankles, first right then left, including the spaces between the toes. The wuḍū' - physical cleansing – is started with the clear intention of focusing attention on the inner aspect of purification. Each stage is sanctified by the recitation of specific passages from the Qur'ān. This purification is followed by Ṣalāh – the most sublime spiritual commencement of the day, which can be offered collectively or individually.[52]

In Ṣalāh, the person stands upright with his face towards the qiblah - the Grand Masjid in the city of Makkah. The consciousness is directed inwards. Both hands are raised gently and then the right hand is placed on the left, just below the navel. This is followed with passages from the Qur'ān. After the recitation and contemplation, the hands are placed on the knees, followed by prostration on the floor. After prostration, there is a period of sitting, accompanied by contemplation and recitation. This is a brief and general sketch of the external process of a profound and powerful form of integrated worship, offered at key intervals throughout the daily cycle. There are a number of stages within Ṣalāh – sublime prayer – focusing the individual's inner self on particular aspects. The process culminates in supplication, the essence and marrow of the whole worship.[53]

Muslim physicians have developed the use of various modes of physical exercise that acts as an effective prophylactic against various diseases, as well as strengthening the body. The wisdom of exercise is profound and far-sighted. It is an established fact that every organism requires food in order to survive and preserve health. However, even if the quality of the food is wholesome and easily assimilable by the body it does leave a certain amount of waste. The eliminative organs try to eliminate waste and toxicity but seldom succeed in clearing all of it. The waste that is left behind gradually accumulates with the potential for disease. The waste and toxins can lead to vitiation and abnormal changes in the general and specific organs, temperament, putrefaction and decay – particularly in the digestive tract – swelling and accumulation and abnormal growths.

It is these and other factors which dictate that steps need to be taken to eliminate waste and toxins. Exercise is one of the most effective and safe ways of eliminating waste products. The use of medication, unless in extreme and serious cases, is to be discouraged. Apart from the elimination of waste products, exercise stimulates the innate heat of the body, making the body stronger and lighter and building up the defences against harmful influences both external and internal. Exercise prevents the accumulation of waste by dispersing and diverting it towards the eliminative organs and channels and assisting in the expulsion of toxins. Thus with sound and regular exercise waste does not accumulate for long periods. The increase of innate heat stimulates the defences, burns out the insidious toxins and strengthens the joints and muscles. The exercise accelerates the absorption of nutrition by the tissues and organs. The organs are expanded and softened, and eliminative organs such as skin pores are dilated. There is an increased intake of oxygen, which in itself purifies and strengthens the entire body.

Exercise can be of two broad kinds: exercise carried out with the clear intention and purpose of benefiting, and exercise incidental to ordinary occupational or life activities. It is the former, proper exercise, which is the subject of our discussion and which wields maximum preventative benefits. The exercise can vary according to its mode, intensity and duration. It may be short or long, mild or strenuous, slow or rapid. It may also be rapid and strenuous or mild and slow. However, moderate exercise is the most suitable.

Strenuous exercises are many, such as wrestling, running, brisk walking, jumping, archery, fencing, and horse riding. The general principle of these strenuous exercises is that they are strong and vigorous. Mild exercises are carriage riding, slow camel-riding, boat cruising, swinging in a lying or sitting position, etc. Bathing in different waters and massage of various types are also forms of cleansing and exercise acting as preventative measures.

There is a suitable exercise for every individual according to his or her specific constitution. Light or mild exercises are appropriate for persons debilitated from diseases such as fever, and who are unable to move about quickly, or cannot stand for long periods. Persons who have used purgatives or are suffering from respiratory conditions such as pleurisy are advised to take mild exercise. The elderly are also recommended these kinds of exercises and the benefits and effects of them are relaxation and sleepiness and dispersion of rīḥ – harmful gases. It helps in poor memory and certain cases of brain damage, stimulates the appetite and helps in conditions of mild depression. Similarly, riding in horse-drawn carriages has beneficial effects but is slightly more potent and may produce shaking of the body. Voyaging and cruising in small vessels close to the coastline is useful for certain speech disorders and skin diseases of dry types. Cruising in deep waters can be beneficial in certain emotional conditions, but it can also generate fear.

Youth and adult life, in general, is the time for strenuous exercise as well as when specific areas need to be strengthened. There are also exercises for individual organs which have particular benefits. For the improvement of eyesight, occasionally gazing at water, green plants and minute objects intently, but without fixing the eyes for too long are some examples. Listening attentively to low-pitched sounds, occasionally interspersed with high-pitched tones helps the hearing. Thus each organ has a range of exercises which aid its function and structure. It is important to bear in mind that there are conditions in which exercise can be harmful and these need to be taken into consideration. The general rules are to protect the weak organs and the weak individual from strenuous exercise. In these cases, exercise needs to be mild. There are some conditions such as varicose veins when movements of the part can be contra-indicated and in such conditions, exercise should be given to the upper parts of the body and the legs rested. In diseases of the cerebral area, the exercise of the head and neck needs to be taken with the advice of a physician. Similarly, for the aged, and for pregnant women, it is advisable to consult a physician before taking systematic exercise.

There are some general rules for exercise of any type. The body needs to be in a state where food has been digested, but not empty. It should be taken at the point when digestion is being replaced with assimilation. Before strenuous exercise, there should be a warming-up period to stimulate the body gently. Massage before any exercise should be with a rough towel and after exercise the sweet oils such as almond oil. The bladder and bowels should be emptied before taking exercise. In hot climates or in summer it is advisable to exercise in the evening. In cold climates or in winter it is advisable to exercise in the morning or during the day. Exercise should be continued as long as the movement of limbs is easy and free. As well as this, the breathing should be such that the person is able to talk. When these signs begin to disappear then exercise should be stopped. The completion of exercising may be followed by a light massage with safe and natural plant oils, such as sweet almond or olive oil. Once a proper schedule of exercise is worked out it should be continued, unless there are reasons to the contrary.

There can be a number of complications from too much or inappropriate exercise which need to be dealt with: there may be dryness, hydration, tightness, fatigue or injury. Hydration can occur in individuals who live a sedentary and rich life, with frequent use of baths and much food. In these cases, there should be dry massage and the recommendation of hard work. Dryness may be caused in an individual with a hot temperament. In such cases rest and gentle massage with oils is the best solution. Flaccidity may be managed with a dry and vigorous massage and by the use of astringent oils. Stiffness is a frequent result of excess exercise, due to the drawing out of toxins from the tissues. Hot baths are helpful along with the application of light oils, moistening foods and rest. In the case of fatigue due to excess or inappropriate exercise, the exercise should be stopped. Recuperative massage which directs the waste towards the skin, together with rest, can also help.

Ghusl – bathing – is a necessary cleansing process which is used extensively in traditional health care. The ḥammāms – or baths of different kinds, were a normal feature in Muslim communities. There was extensive use of them by all sections of the community as preventative and curative aids. The particular benefits of bathing are induction of sleep, cleansing of the skin, removal of fatigue, dispersal of waste matters and drawing of blood towards the skin. Of course, indiscriminate or inappropriate use of bathing can be injurious. Excessive use may weaken the heart, produce nausea and fainting and disturb stagnate matter. General guidance with regard to bathing is to consider the season, the time of day, and the condition of the stomach. Cold baths are most suitable in summer and in hot climates, whereas warm baths should be used in winter and in cold regions. Cold baths should be avoided by weak, dyspeptic and catarrhal individuals.

Community Health Measures

Earlier in this chapter the Islamic approach to the spiritual and hygienic needs of an individual was illustrated. The balanced nature of the Islamic way of life is such that it deals with the community and has a collective dimension. Indeed, the term ummah - used to describe Muslims – means 'community'. The emphasis on communal life is an Islamic approach. The individual can only develop within a harmonious, integrated and well-knit community. From the early inception of the community in Madīnah, the Prophet ﷺ regulated and paid attention to health and hygiene. The cleanliness and promotion of specific and general matters of community health constitute an important aspect of Islamic medicine. The Prophet ﷺ dealt with issues of contagion and infection. About plagues, he said:

> "*If you hear it has infected a certain area, stay away from it. But if it infects an area you happen to be in, do not move away from it to escape the disease.*" [54]

These and many other principles and practices were used in the formulation of community health policies and the organisation of environmental health. One of the central concepts and practices is the ṭahārah – purification.[55] The Islamic classic medical texts deal with community health under separate studies referred to as ḥifẓ aṣ-ṣiḥḥah – 'The Maintenance of Health'. The matters of sanitation, the quality and sources of water, the burial of the dead and other collective aspects of health are dealt with in considerable detail. Indeed there is advice to individuals attending collective prayer to refrain from eating raw onions and garlic and to use perfumes whilst attending community functions. It is this Islamic emphasis when practised and actualised, which enabled healthy and ecologically safe communities and the wider environment.

FASTING: AN INSTITUTION FOR HEALTH PROMOTION

Ṣawm – complete fasting – is one institution that meets spiritual, physical, individual and community needs in a most harmonious way. The spiritual aspect of an individual is developed and enhanced in the most potent and sublime manner. Taqwā – God-consciousness, discipline, and empathy with the poor and needy – is the main emphasis behind fasting. As a devotional process, and for internal purification, fasting enables the person to transcend his gross physical needs. The deep cleansing process clears the mind and the internal organs and tissue. Biologically, fasting is an effective, natural process of detoxification and healing. Voluntary fasting is an intensely personal process. However, the manner of fasting in the Islamic tradition is a community affair.

The period of community-regulated fasting is the month of Ramadan each year. The fact that the Islamic community uses a lunar calendar gives dynamism to the whole process. The months rotate according to the various seasons over the period. The four seasons of the year change from one season to another. Thus, the individual enjoys the spiritual and physical benefits both preventative and curative at different periods. This timing itself indicates the natural and dynamic adaptability of the Islamic health tradition to the needs of individuals and communities over time and space.

Fasting is a potent process. This fact must be taken into account and certain basic precautions should be noted. Children under the age of puberty are advised not to fast. Men and women who are old or have serious diseases need to consult a physician before embarking on the fast. Pregnant or lactating women and also travellers need to be cautious and would be advised not to fast.[56]

8

Principles of Treatment

"*Within the human being there is a morsel of flesh, and when it is corrupt, the body is corrupt, and when it is sound, the body is sound. Truly it is the* qalb *(heart).*"

The Prophet Muhammad ﷺ

Management of Essential Factors

Treatment in traditional Islamic medicine consists of a number of different therapies selected and adapted to both the general and specific needs of the individual patient. The various levels of treatment are management of essential factors, use of medicaments, psycho-spiritual healing, manipulative measures and surgical intervention. The management of essential factors which was discussed in the chapter on pathogenesis provides broad options capable of restoring balance without the use of medicaments. Management of the 'six essentials', as they are sometimes known, consists of suitable modification. Food, one of these factors, can be considered to illustrate this, using general principles for managing the quality and quantity of food as a therapeutic measure. Ṭibb nutrition is based on the concept that for each food, whether it is fruit, vegetable or meat, there is an energetic quality. This framework of the four primary qualities, as they apply to various foods, enables the physician to tailor dietary recommendations, in a holistic manner and context, to the individual's temperament or particular imbalance.

In nutritional therapy, food can be withheld, increased, or given in moderate quantity, depending upon the needs and conditions of the individual patient and the nature of the disease. Food serves to provide energy and replaces the loss that results from the various activities of life and living. From an Islamic perspective, there are interconnections between food and the states of consciousness and emotional processes. In any disease, there is an imbalance that also disturbs the various aspects of a person. The fact that an individual is considered one dynamic and integrated whole helps us to see the interconnections. Food is one of the most potent and yet safe instruments for establishing balance in a disturbed organism. Each individual ingredient in the diet is studied and understood in the holistic conceptual and empirical framework which was discussed in earlier chapters. The Ḥakīms classify ranges of foods on their qualitative basis of hot or cold, and dry or moist. The qualitative natures of foods are part and parcel of common knowledge and folk traditions within Islamic communities. Traditionally, the selection of foods is based on the season, age and needs of the individual. The therapeutic use of foods consists of using qualitative understanding and quantity in a sensitive and controlled manner. A diet consisting mainly of fruit and vegetables is different in quality from, for example, a diet of half-boiled eggs and meats. Individuals with hot diseases such as fevers need essentially to use cooling, leafy vegetables. Individuals with a good appetite but immature Humours should be encouraged to change to a bulky diet. This will satisfy the appetite without adding to the quantity of the Humours.

The quantity of food is generally reduced or stopped in acute disease and sometimes chronic conditions. In chronic conditions, strength and vitality have been lost for a considerable time and have to be maintained by the supply of food. In acute diseases, however, it is expected that the strength of the patient will be sufficient for their body to respond to the diseased condition with a healing crisis, culminating in health. The regulation of food at the critical stage of the disease, when the vital force is actively engaged in the struggle, requires a light diet. Indeed, the more acute the illness and the nearer the time of the crisis, the lighter the food should be, unless there are contraindications.

Other factors in food management which are taken into consideration are the rate of digestion and absorption of foods. Heavy and viscid foods such as beef are avoided in cases of stasis and obstruction. Assimilable and energy-giving foods such as honey are included when there is such a need in conditions following prolonged illness. The psychological states and physiological conditions of an individual are also important considerations. The symbolic relationship of foods derived from cultural and religious sources must also be taken into account when planning any food therapy with an individual patient.

TREATMENT THROUGH A SINGLE REMEDY

In Islamic medicine, there is a distinction between medicaments that are mufradāt – single, and medicaments that are murakkabāt – compound.[57] The traditional use of an individual substance in the treatment of various diseases still continues to be practised as a therapy of choice today. The range of substances used in the alleviation of suffering reflects the wide range of the richness that exists in Nature's treasury. Remedies may be used from the mineral, plant and animal kingdoms, and in practice, most remedies come from plant sources. In treatment, the principle that each human being is a reflection of all creation is followed by using a whole range of substances. Thus the analogy of micro-macro constitutes a biological reality and also has application in medical practice.[58] The use of a single remedy is based on sound theoretical foundations and is supported by observations and experiments of countless generations of reputable physicians. Such empirical knowledge and wisdom, particularly in pharmacognosy, is considerable and constitutes important skills in Islamic medical practice. The general emphasis in planning medicament therapy is to re-establish the lost balance within an individual patient with minimum intervention and change. The medicaments are used and selected after meticulous and comprehensive life history, with particular reference to the medical aspects of an individual patient in the context of their family. The remedies are used in an active biological state rather than isolating a specific chemically or pharmacologically active element. The physician has to know each specific remedy in full detail. The physician must know the:

- Name of the remedy;
- Identification and study of its natural habitat;
- Nature of the remedy;
- Specific energy pattern;
- Physiochemical actions;
- Indications of its uses in general and specific conditions;
- Specific relationship to organs;
- Duration of its action;
- Toxicity and contra-indications;
- Types of preparation;
- Dosage, administration and antidote.

The modes of administration are many, depending on factors such as the nature of the disease, organ, etc. The general principle is to use medicine in a condition that is effective but without any harmful side effects. There are a range of preparations such as infusions, decoctions, tinctures, extracts, tablets, pills, elixirs, electuaries and oils, with ointments and creams for external applications. The whole range of different parts of plants are used including roots, rhizomes, stems, barks, leaves, flowers, gums and oils.

The selection of a remedy depends upon the understanding and evaluation of an individual patient's temperament, the nature, severity and location of the disease. The physician also has to consider the sex, age, season, lifestyle, residence, occupation and previous treatment of the individual patient. Each of the above factors has to be applied in order to restore the lost or displaced equilibrium. An imbalanced organ provides an illustrative example. If the practitioner considers that an organ is diseased, then whilst paying attention to the other factors he has to select a single medicine with regard to the temperament of the organ affected, its structure, position and vitality.

Temperament is the energy pattern of the organ and provides information of the highest importance. When the original and normal energy pattern of the affected organ is known, it is relatively easy for the practitioner to assess the extent of abnormality, and the appropriate dosage and potency of the remedy. If the affected organ is of hot temperament whilst the disease is cold, it indicates a gross abnormality which will require strong doses. However, if the original temperament is cold and the disease is also of the same quality then mild doses will re-establish the lost balance. The position and the relationships of the affected organ are important too. Anatomical knowledge is helpful in the selection of the mode of administration of a remedy. The position of an organ can give an indication of the accessibility of an organ for remedial action. For example, the stomach is more easily influenced by mild medicament than the lungs. Each organ has interrelationships with other organs which help in determining treatment. The relationship of the liver to the kidneys and stomach is a useful example. If there is morbid matter in the upper part of the liver it can easily be eliminated through the kidneys, whereas if it is in the lower part of the liver it is better disposed of through the bowels. Correspondingly, the structure of an organ will give information which will indicate the level of penetration and absorption. Spongy organs respond differently to medicine, compared with solid ones. The vitality of an organ is a significant factor in planning any treatment. The fundamental or vital organs such as the heart, brain, and liver need milder medicine, as any disturbance or too rapid change can cause serious complications. The vitality of an organ can also give an indication of the level of morbid matter and toxicity. Sensitivity and the normal function of the organ also have to be considered in the selection of a single remedy so as to avoid irritation or possible injurious effects.

Use of Compound Medicines

The use of compound medicaments is also employed in the treatment of internal diseases of complex and chronic nature. In traditional Islamic medicine, although the general preference is for a single remedy, there are diseases in which using more than one substance combined in a coherent way and on a thought-out basis enables a speedier cure. There are certain medicines which when used singly, even if in limited amounts, have certain undesirable side effects. Muslim practitioners developed this branch of art and published authoritative works such as *Aqrabadin – Pharmacopeia.* The classical Greek and Indian sources were particularly utilised in the development of the use of compounds by Muslim physicians and continued to be prepared and manufactured in the traditional methods by individual practitioners and natural medicine companies.[59] Works by masters of Islamic medicine such as Ibn Sīnā and Rāzī continue to be used as basic reference by today's practitioners of traditional Ṭibb. With the emergence of new stresses, deficiencies and patterns of disease, there are formulations which take into account the new conditions. Generally, only reputable Ḥakīms' formulations are used. Usually the formulation of compound remedies, or change in any traditional forms, is a complicated process requiring deep understanding of Materia Medica, and of human diseases, as well as considerable experience.

The Use of the Qur'an in Healing

An essential feature of the philosophy and practice of Islamic medicine is its harmony and ability to respond to the total needs of human beings. Islamic medicine has many facets which, on the one hand, relate to physical needs, and on the other hand, are intimately bound with the higher order, and are responsive to the intangible aspects of the person. The whole phenomenon of creation is one that has the potential of uplifting and promoting creativity as well as the ability to degrade and debase. The existence and influence of destructive forces are also acknowledged, in particular the causes of insidious diseases of psycho-spiritual origin.

The Qur'ān depicts this reality in vivid language in a number of places:

> "*Say: I seek refuge in the Lord of the Daybreak,*
> *from the evil of what he has created;*
> *from the evil of darkness when it gathers;*
> *from the evil of conjuring witches;*
> *from the evil of the envier when he envies.*"
>
> (Sūrat al-Falaq)

This awareness and understanding of the cosmological situation has enabled the Ḥakīms to respond to diseases requiring intervention on a higher level. The Islamic Sharī'ah – Divine Law – prohibits the practice and use of siḥr – magic – in treatment. The Qur'ān in its totality and certain sections and verses in particular, is curative of serious conditions not amenable to other forms of treatment.[60] Muslim physicians use guidance and specific verses from the Qur'ān in treatment. There are many methods in which specific verses of the Qur'ān are used in a particular sequence and recited:

- Ta'wīdh – literally meaning 'refuge' – in which sections of the Qu'rān are used;
- Da'wah – invocation;
- Ruqyā – 'charms'.[61]

Surgical Intervention

Surgery has been an integral part of the practice and study of traditional Islamic medicine. Physicians were trained both in surgery and internal medicine. It was during Abū'l-Qāsim az-Zahrāwī's time that the practice of surgery reached its zenith. His classical work on the art, *Kitāb at-Taṣrīf – The Method of Medicine* – dealt with the subject in detail. Az-Zahrāwī for the first time in history drew each instrument in colour.

The general misunderstanding, namely that controlled dissection of the human body in the Islamic community prevents the growth and development of anatomical and physiological knowledge, is inaccurate. The study of the human form has been an important aspect of Muslim scholarship to the extent that philosophers and mystics like al-Ghazālī thought it important in their Gnostic traditions. Indeed, physicians and surgeons, for instance, Ibn Nafīs, were aware of the lesser circulation in 687 A.H. (1288 C.E.).[62] Muslim surgeons used and developed a wide range of surgical instruments which were not only useful but beautiful and artistic in their looks. There were a number of surgical procedures that were used, from Caesarean section to complicated eye operations. The Muslim surgeon Thābit ibn Quraah was using tanwīn – anaesthesia - in operations of the eyes as early as 850 A.H. (1492 C.E).[63] The present situation in traditional Islamic medicine schools, unfortunately, does not reflect this outstanding surgical knowledge. Since colonial subjugation, in particular, the level of knowledge and skills of Ḥakīms in surgery declined to such an extent that it may be said to be non-existent.[64]

9

THE FUTURE OF ISLAMIC MEDICINE

" *We will soon show them Our signs in the Universe and in their own souls, until it will become quite clear to them that it is the truth. Is not sufficient as regards your Lord that He is witness over all things? Now surely they are in doubt as to the meeting of their Lord; now surely He encompasses all things.* "

(Sūrah Fuṣṣilat, āyat 53-54)

SOCIO-CULTURAL IMPLICATIONS

In this final chapter, the focus will be to consider the future role of the Islamic healthcare tradition for health, well-being, and its socio-cultural, economic and peace implications and benefits. Of course, these considerations do not constitute part of the accepted body of Islamic medical knowledge.

Given the prohibitive cost of technologically-based medicine, its inability to cure increasing chronic diseases and the rising dissatisfaction - to the point of alienation - on the part of the intelligent public, a positive and important future is indicated for Islamic medicine.[65] Its holistic and liberating paradigms along with clinical and therapeutic experiences, along with a gentle, efficacious, and rich treasury of natural medicaments, places Islamic medicine as a medicine of the future.

It is surprising to what extent a tradition of healthcare with such positive characteristics as Islamic medicine has been hidden and ignored, and it would perhaps be helpful to consider why this has happened to such an economical and natural form of medicine.

The breakdown of Islamic culture was followed by subjugation and colonial domination. The colonial powers successfully disintegrated and fragmented most of the remaining Muslim societies. This physical disintegration was followed by the destruction of economic, political and socio-cultural and scientific structures. The traditional colleges of Islamic medicine, hospitals and professional organisations were systemically deprived of essential resources and freedom to practice and develop. The status and positive images of the Ḥakīms and Ṭabībs – physicians, were degraded. In a number of countries in the Muslim world, their practices and teachings were made unlawful.[66]

However, the grassroots popularity of Islamic medicine and its appeal and practical usefulness, enables it to be practised in various forms. Its practice and teaching were well-organised and deep-rooted in India, Bangladesh, Malaysia and Pakistan.[67] The political independence of Muslim lands has been accompanied by increasing awareness of cultural and scientific traditions and heritage. The Islamic reconstruction has also begun to give prominence to Islamic sciences, including medicine.[68] The need for appropriate and effective medical care for masses of people provides new impetus for the future of Islamic medicine.

Economic Considerations

Today, the practice of medicine is a major economic enterprise. The medical industry of our time is one of the largest and most powerful, particularly the multinational pharmaceutical companies. The mechanistic approach of the dominant medical schools has led to a huge and cumbersome technological industry for diagnosis and treatment which knows no limits. Within the industrialised nations of Europe and the United States of America, there is increasing dissatisfaction with high-technology methods which alienate patients from their practitioners. The human dimension of care and sensitivity has been replaced by intrusive and insidious machines. Medical technology and pharmaceutical drugs sap away major chunks of the healthcare budget. The toxic side effects of pharmaceutical drugs and most forms of mechanical diagnosis are becoming a health menace. Government and research scholars are beginning to alert the public to the economically unsuitable health service and there is now a serious re-assessment of the whole basis of health care.[69] Indeed there is tremendous interest in, and growth of, human-oriented and economical health alternatives within most industrialised nations. Given these considerations, it is important that non-industrialised nations maintain and develop traditional healthcare resources.

TOWARDS HEALTH, HAPPINESS AND PEACE

The present age can be appropriately said to be the age of tranquillisers and violence. Each day some new tranquilliser is invented and introduced into the already extensive toxic armoury of chemical drugs, promising the ever-elusive state of peace and tranquillity. However, the range and level of mental and emotional disturbances and diseases are on the increase. The manifold stress of industrial life, a toxic environment and subversive, drug-based medicines compound the agony and suffering towards insanity and complete disintegration of the core of human beings. Highly mechanised hospitals with numerous specialists themselves appear to be victims of the process of dehumanisation by modern technocratic medicine. It is in this desperate context that Islamic medicine can provide primordial wisdom, healing, and creative energy with its gentle and effective treasury of natural medicine. The agonised and suffering masses could benefit enormously through the holistic and natural tradition of Islamic medicine. It is the benevolent Creator who has created relief for mankind through His mercy and love. True health, peace and happiness come through unification with the Truth.

GLOSSARY

Akhlāt	The four Humours: Blood, Phlegm, Yellow Bile and Black Bile. These constitute the biological basis of Islamic medicine.
ʿaql	An apprehending light, unique to human beings, that guides the individual towards balanced decisions and actions.
Aqrabadin	A pharmacopoeia of compound medicine, giving details of individual substances and directions for their manufacture and use.
Arkān	The four basic Elements: Fire, Air, Water and Earth.
āyah	A Qur'ānic term which means signs and manifestations, which, when reflected upon, guide towards purpose and meaning.
Bayt al-Ḥikmah	The House of Wisdom, an academy founded in Baghdad by the Abbasids to promote the systemic research and development of sciences.
Bimāristān	A place for the sick, a hospital.

Bulghum	Phlegm, one of the four Humours, associated with the Element Water, being cold and moist in nature.
diyah	Blood money paid in compensation for a homicide.
dīn al-fiṭrah	The primordial tradition and way of life, Islam.
ghayb	The hidden or unseen aspect of existence which beyond normal human sensory perception.
Ḥakīm	An individual endowed with knowledge experience and wisdom, a sage. The title is given to a consultant physician of Islamic medicine.
ḥalāl	Lawful and permitted food, nutrition and behaviour which is life giving.
ḥammān	A bath, generally deep cleansing, alternatingly warm and cold.
ḥarām	Opposite of ḥalāl, unlawful, destructive nutrition or behaviour.

ḥifz aṣ-ṣiḥaḥ	Hygiene and public health matters with emphasis on prevention of ill health.
iʿtidāl	A dynamic condition of balance and equilibrium.
jism	The material body.
khamr	Intoxicant; that which covers up the reason; alcohol.
laṭīf	Subtle and penetrative force.
miswāk	A traditional root, used from the time of the Prophet Muḥammad ﷺ.
mufradāt	Individual drugs, usually of plant origin, in their natural states, or: a class of traditional Islamic medical literature, which deals with the study and uses of natural substances.
murakkabāt	Compound medicines, prepared from a number of individual substances, or: a class of Islamic medical texts dealing with the use and manufacture of compound medicines.

mizāj	A dynamic functional state which reflects the energy pattern of an individual person or thing.
nafs	The self, which can be in a number of states: an-nafs al-ammārah – fossilised and insensitive; an-nafs al-lawwāmah – reproachful and agitated; an-nafs al-muṭma'innah – tranquil or balanced.
qalb	The 'heart'; an immaterial principle which regulates the predominantly psycho-emotional life of a person.
rīḥ	A harmful type of gaseous wind, usually in the stomach.
rūḥ	The vital force, a purposeful and dynamic force that permeates the human organism. It has different names, depending on its function and location: ḥaywāniyyah – centred in the heart and maintains life; nafsāniyyah – located in the brain and promotes sensation in movement; and ṭabayyah – located in the liver, for the preservation of the individual, and in the

	ovaries and testicles, for the preservation of the species.
Rūḥ	The spirit which is of divine origin and is transcendental.
Ṣafrā	Yellow Bile, one of the four Humours corresponding to the Element Fire, and hot and dry in its qualities.
sakīnah	A state of peace and tranquillity; the result of unification with the truth.
Saudā	Black Bile, one of the four Humours, corresponding to the Element Earth and cold and dry in its qualities.
sharī'ah	A path, paradigm of principles and practices which enables human beings to live in harmony with reality.
ṭahārah	Purity and cleanliness of an individual and community.
taqwā	A state in consciousness which guides one to refrain from destructive behaviour.

Ṭibb	Literally means 'nature'; refers to holistic medicine.
Ṭibb an-Nabawī	'The Medicine of the Prophet ﷺ', or Prophetic medicine.
waḥi	Divine Revelation which is direct knowledge from The Creator.
ẓāhir	The external or outward aspects of creation and existence.

Notes & References

Historical Background

[1] T. P. Hughes, *Dictionary of Islam,* Cosmos Publications, New Delhi, 1978, p. 17.

[2] N. Groom, *Frankincense and Myrrh,* Longman, London, 1981, p. 96.

[3] Hughes, op. cit., p. 18.

[4] Sūrat an-Najm, āyāt 19–20. Qur'ānic references are quoted in this format, which refers to the Sūrah – chapter, as it is known in Arabic, followed by the number of the āyah – sign, which is equivalent to verse or sentence, in this case.

[5] A. A. Maududi, *The Philosophy of Hajj,* Idara Tarjuman-ul-Quran, Lahore, 1976, p. 20.

[6] Sayyid Qutb, *In the Shade of the Qu'rān,* Muslim Welfare House Publishers, London, 1979, p. 66.

[7] M. B. Badri, *Islam and Alcoholism,* American Trust Publications, London, 1978, p. 11.

[8] Ibid. p. 11.

[9] Ibid. p. 9.

[10] Ibid. p. 12.

[11] M. Ullman, *Islamic Medicine*, Edinburgh University Press, 1978, p. 1.

[12] As-Suyūtī, *Ṭibb an-Nabī*, Osiris, 1962, Vol. 4, p. 51.

[13] S. H. H. Nadvi, *Medical Philosophy in Islam and Contribution of Muslim in the Advancement of Medical Sciences*, Academia, University of Durban, Durban, 1983, p. 7.

[14] C. Elgood, *A Medical History of Persia and the Eastern Caliphate*, Cambridge University Press, 1951, p. 49.

[15] Ibid. p. 49.

[16] E. G. Browne, *Arabian Medicine*, Cambridge University Press, 1962, p. 15.

[17] M. Z. Siddiqi, *Studies in Arabic and Persian Medical Literature*, Calcutta University, 1959, p. 24.

[18] S. H. Nasr, *Islamic Science*, World of Islam Festival Publishing co. London 1976, p. 187.

[19] Ibid. p. 189.

[20] A word of Persian origin combining vimār – meaning sick and stān – meaning place. The word literally means hospital.

[21] Elgood, op. cit,. p. 70.

[22] Ibid. p. 76.

[23] Ibid. p. 175.

[24] M. H. Shah, *The General Principles of Avicenna's Canon of Medicine*, Naveed Clinic, Karachi, 1966, p. 439.

[25] Nasr op.cit., p. 187.

[26] S. H. Nasr, *Science and Civilisation in Islam*, Harvard University Press, 1968, p. 213.

[27] M. Said, *Hamard Medical Digest*, 1959, Vol 1-2, p. 136.

[28] Personal communication and discussion with Ḥakīm Muḥammad Nabi Khān and Ḥakīm Muḥammad Riaz Qersih Ṣāḥib, may Allah have mercy upon them.

PHILOSOPHICAL CONCEPTIONS OF ISLAMIC MEDICINE

[29] The essential philosophical concepts are derived from the Qur'ān, the Ḥadith – traditions and sayings of the Prophet ﷺ – and the works of Islamic scholars such as al-Ghazālī and Ibn ʿArabī.

[30] S. H. Nasr, *An Introduction to Islamic Cosmological Doctrines*, Thames and Hudson, London, 1978, pp. 101-102.

[31] Ibn Sīnā, *The Principle of Medicine*, Naveed Clinic, Karachi, 1966, p. 142.

[32] S. H. Nasr, *Science and Civilisation in Islam*, Harvard University Press, 1968, p. 184.

THE PSYCHOLOGICAL FOUNDATIONS

[33] Al-Gazālī, *Kimya-I-Sadat*, Sheikh Ghulam Ali & Sons, Lahore, 1977, p. 60.

[34] Sūrat al-Fajr, āyah 27.

[35] Sūrat al-Qiyāmah, āyah 2.

[36] Sūrat Yūsuf, āyah 53.

[37] Ibn Sīnā, *Kitāb al-Adwiyā al-Qalbiyah*, Iran Society, Calcutta, 1956, p. 1.

PHYSIOLOGICAL CONCEPTS

[38] Quwwah – energy is a central concept in Islamic medicine.

[39] O.C. Gruner, *The Cannon of Medicine of Avicenna,* Augustus M. Kelly, New York 1970, p. 34.

[40] Ibid., p. 35.

[41] This is the classical way of studying anatomy and physiology.

LIFE BALANCE

[42] One can see the holistic nature of Islamic medicine, in that it takes account of the multifarious factors acting and reacting upon an individual.

[43] M. H. Shah, *The General Principles of Avicenna's Canon of Medicine*, Naveed Clinic, Karachi, 1966, p. 156.

[44] The water of Zamzam occupies a special curative and preventative place in Islamic medicine. One of the characteristics of Zamzam is that it is not subject to putrefaction like other waters.

[45] The preventative measures can be rightly referred to as ecological adaptations. The modern speciality of clinical ecology is a rediscovery of the wider principles illustrated in this chapter. See R. Mackarness, *Chemical Victims*, Pan, London, 1980, pp. 1-20.

DIAGNOSIS

[46] These are the indications of health and balance, see O.C. Gruner, *The Canon of Medicine of Avicenna,* Augustus M. Kelley, New York, 1970, pp. 381-456.

[47] The central clinical concept in Islamic Medicine is that of Mizāj – temperament; evaluation of energy patterns.

[48] I am grateful to Ḥakīm Nūr Muḥammad Hani for his help in the study of pulse diagnosis.

[49] Gruner, op. cit., pp. 323-346.

[50] Ibid., p. 355.

PREVENTATIVE ASPECTS

[51] The Latin name of the particular tree is *Salvadora persica,* whose preventative and curative value has been studied analytically in Switzerland by Pharba Basle Ltd.

[52] Al-Ghazālī, *Kimya-l-Sadat*, Sheikh Ghulam Ali & Sons, Lahore, 1977, pp. 164–183.

[53] Al-Ghazālī, *Kimya-l-Sadat*, Sheikh Ghulam Ali & Sons, Lahore, 1977, p. 231. The source of this is Bukhārī.

[54] Al-Bukhārī, *Ṣāḥīḥ al-Bukhārī*, Vol. 7, Dār al-Fikr, Makkah, pp. 418–420.

[55] Sūrat al-Baqarah, āyah 222.

[56] The Sharīʿah and traditions of the Prophet Muḥammad صلى الله عليه وسلم, specifically advise for people in these categories to not fast.

PRINCIPLES OF TREATMENT

[57] This is a classical division of Materia Medica by Muslim physicians and scholars

[58] The research in our own age is also moving towards this realisation that human beings contain the different energies and physiochemical constituents of the Earth, as well as the different forces.

[59] Dāwakhānāh Ḥakīm Ajmal Khān Ltd. of Lahore, *Methods of Medicaments Preparations.*

[60] Sūrah Tāāhār, āyah 69.

[61] A. Ali, *Amal-I-Qurani*, Naz Publishing House, Delhi p. 15.

[62] S. H. Nasr, *Science and Civilization in Islam,* Harvard University Press, 1969, p. 213.

[63] M. Bayrakdar, 'The First Use of Anaesthesia', *Imam*, 1984, pp. 52-53.

[64] The reasons are many for this situation, with the most apparent being that the governments is reluctant to fund surgery in traditional colleges as well as the Ḥakīms' own lack of surgical skills

THE FUTURE OF ISLAMIC MEDICINE

[65] S. Fulder and R. Monr, *The Status of Complementary Medicine,* The Threshold Foundation, London, 1981, pp. 1-19. This and many other reports and publications indicate the need for holistic health care.

[66] In parts of the Arabian Peninsula even today Ḥakīms are not allowed to practice or set up professional organisations.

[67] India and Pakistan are the leading pioneers in promoting Islamic Medicine with central and regional government funding.

[68] The Islamic Medicine Organisation (I.M.O) in Kuwait is an example, as well as the work of Ḥakīm Muḥammad Saʿīd, President of the Hamdard Foundation in Karachi, Pakistan. See also Z. Sardar, *Science and Technology in the Middle East,* Longman, London, 1982, pp. 18–23.

[69] I. Kennedy, *The Unmasking of Medicine,* George Allen & Unwin, London, 1981, pp. 117–169.

Selected Prophetic Recipes and Ingredients for Maintaining and Improving Health and Wellbeing

" *We have sent among you an apostle Muhammad* (صلى الله عليه وسلم) *from among yourselves, rehearsing to you our signs and instructing you in scripture and wisdom and in new knowledge.*"

(Sūrat al-Baqarah, āyah 150)

Throughout the life of the Prophet Muhammad صلى الله عليه وسلم, many healing ingredients were emphasised in their blessed teachings and practices, including a number that were identified in Divine revelation.

Here is a small selection of Prophetic recipes and ingredients, and some insights into their invaluable potential for helping to maintain and improve health and wellbeing.

The next few pages will introduce the following six items:

- Talbīna – Prophetic Barley Porridge
- Nabīdh – Prophetic Health Drink
- Raisins – The Royal Fruit
- Water – Source of Life and Vitality
- Black Seed – The Blessed Seed
- Honey – The Complete Food and Remedy

Talbīna – Prophetic Barley Porridge – Benefits

Talbīna – barley porridge is a nourishing Prophetic breakfast. Barley is recognised as a sacred and blessed grain in various traditions. Prophet Muhammad ﷺ said: "It removes the grief of the patient's heart, removes its weakness as you remove the dirt from your face after washing it".

It is a perfect food that is high in fibre, particularly soluble fibre. It is high in minerals such as calcium, magnesium, potassium and iron. Talbīna may help with the following: removing constipation, helping people with diabetes, improving heart health, and removing sadness and depression.

Talbīna – Prophetic Barley Porridge – Method

1. Take organic pot barley and dry roast it.

2. Place 7 tablespoons (100g) of the roasted barley in a pan, and add 300ml of water. Heat and simmer for 30 minutes (or until it is cooked and soft), stirring occasionally.

3. Add 100ml of raw milk (organic is ideal) and bring to a boil.

4. After it has cooled. Serve with raw organic honey to taste.

TALBĪNA – VARIATIONS AND TIPS

• You may use a dairy-free alternative such as almond milk. If you do this, add it at the end when serving, not while cooking.

• For extra flavour and nourishment, you may wish to add any of the following: pure tahini, almond butter, and chopped pitted dates.

• You may add black seed paste to help with immune support.

• While roasting the barley, you may wish to add some olive oil.

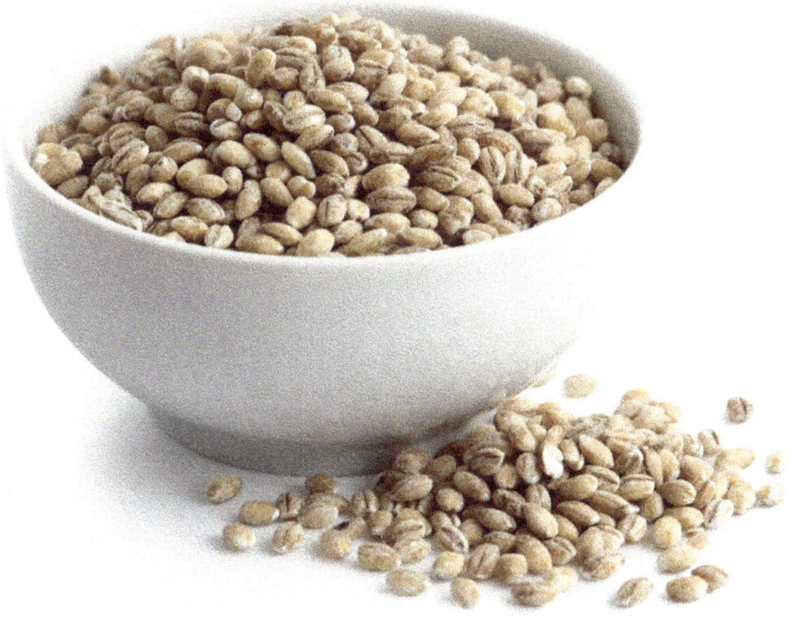

NABĪDH – PROPHETIC HEALTH DRINK – BENEFITS

"*If somebody takes seven ajwa dates in the morning, neither magic nor poison will hurt him that day.*" The Prophet Muhammad ﷺ

The date tree has been mentioned twenty times in the Qur'ān, more than any other fruit. Dates are generally very nutritive and energising, and so they help to gain weight. They can help against heart problems, stomach problems, and sexual weakness. The seeds of ajwa dates are used as a remedy for diabetes. Dates are rich in many vitamins and minerals including calcium, iron, potassium and magnesium. They are also a source of protein and fibre.

Nabīdh is a Prophetic health drink. This nutritious drink gives you the benefits of dates as well as water. It can be used to help with energy, especially after fasting, and to remedy constipation.

NABĪDH – PROPHETIC HEALTH DRINK – METHOD

1. Soak 100g of dates (pitted, which means with pits removed) in 1 litre of pure clean water. Cover and leave overnight.

2. In the morning, blend the mixture to obtain a beautiful cloudy Nabīdh. Drink within 12 hours.

CAUTION: Do not leave Nabīdh for longer than 12 hours or it will ferment and become alcoholic, especially in hot climates.

Nabīdh – Prophetic Health Drink – Variations and Tips

• People with a cool or cold temperament can add ¼ tsp of cinnamon or ginger powder to their Nabīdh drink.

• You can choose to use 100g of raisins instead of dates. However, do not mix dates and raisins, only use one.

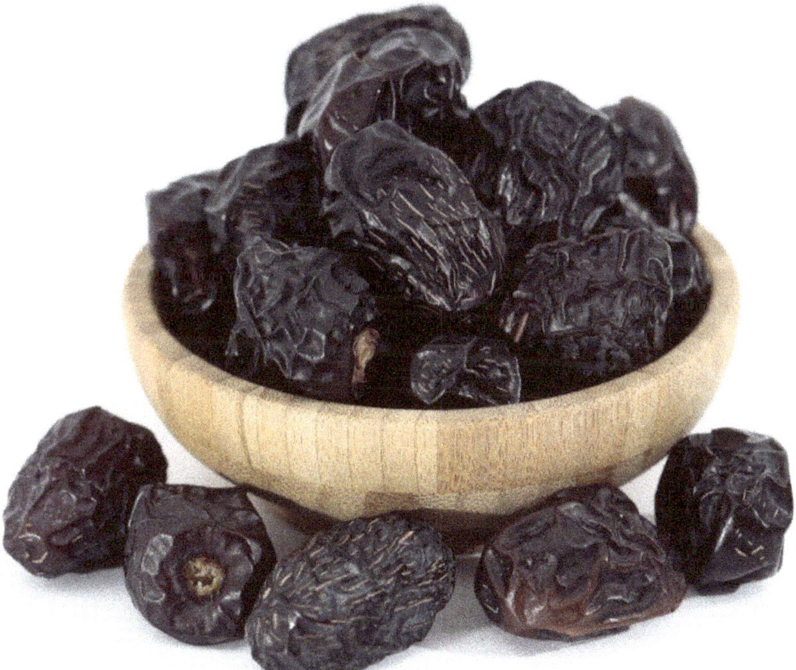

RAISINS – THE ROYAL FRUIT

"*How good are raisins! They remove fatigue, strengthen nerves, extinguish anger, clarify the complexion and sweeten the breath.*"

Human civilisations since time immemorial have used – and often abused – grapes and their products. From a health maintenance point of view, raisins are more useful than grapes.

A product of grape cultivation dating back to 5000 B.C.E., raisins are renowned for their rejuvenating properties. The Qur'ān mentions this fruit eleven times. Raisins are traditionally known as one of the three 'royal fruits' along with dates and figs.

Energetically, raisins are hot and moist. They are used for nourishing and strengthening the body, especially the heart and the digestive system. They can help in treating fevers, coughs, catarrh, jaundice and sub-acute cases of enlarged liver and spleen.

Raisins are nutrient-dense super-foods. They are rich in potassium, magnesium, calcium, phosphorous, manganese, iron, and copper. They also contain fructose, a natural sugar easily absorbed by the body, as well as vitamins A, C, and some B vitamins. Resveratrol, also found in raisins, has been heralded as a 'fountain of youth'.

" *When I travelled the world to find the health secrets of the oldest people, I discovered most of them lived where grapes grow best.*"

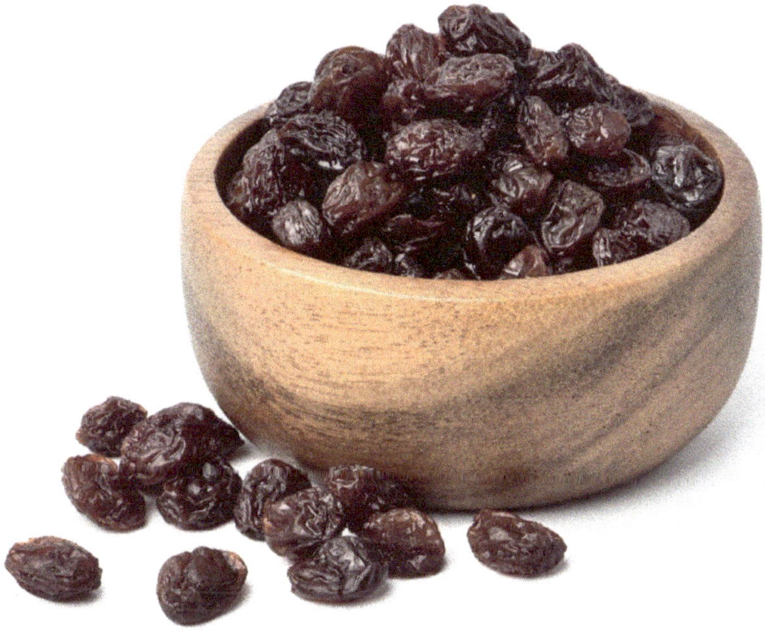

WATER – SOURCE OF LIFE AND VITALITY

"*And we made every living thing of Water.*"

(Sūrat al-'Anbyā', āyah 30)

The adult human body is 60% water, while the Earth's surface is about 70% water. Water is cold and moist energetically. It stimulates appetite, aids digestion, moisturises, and invigorates. Its importance is deeply rooted in all healthcare traditions, including Tibb, with its correct use being crucial for maintaining health.

Water that is sourced from a natural spring is preferred, ideally from a pristine and unpolluted environment such as the mountains.

Required water intake varies depending on temperament. Seasonal changes, occupation, gender, diet and physical activity are also factors. Those factors which increase heat and dryness in the individual will also increase the individual's need for water.

Water is best consumed away from main meals. Watermelon and melon should not be consumed alongside water. Avoid iced or chilled water, especially for those with a cold temperament.

The Prophetic etiquette for drinking water is sitting, taking three measured intakes, with a breath taken in between each one.

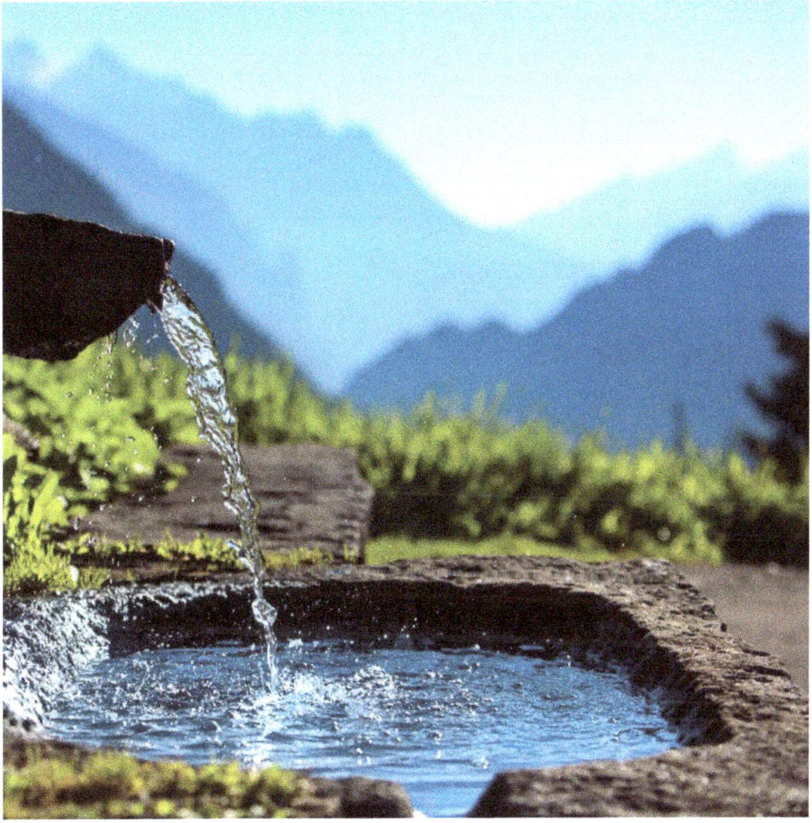

Black Seed – The Blessed Seed

" *This black seed is healing for all diseases except death.*"

The Prophet Muhammad ﷺ

Nigella sativa, black seed or black cumin, is a plant producing an aromatic seed that has a sharp, spicy, and somewhat bitter taste. This seed has held a significant role, including references in the Torah and the Bible. The properties of the black seed are so varied and effective that it has been seen as a miracle cure throughout history.

Black seed, being energetically hot and dry, can support metabolism and digestion, and lowering blood sugar. Black seed has the ability to uplift the mood, hence it has been described as a 'glance of light'.

Black seed oil is abundant in amino acids, phosphorus, iron, carotene, albumin, and antioxidants, bolstering the body's natural healing processes and immune system. It is used as both a preventative and treatment mechanism for various ailments.

To use whole black seeds, take 1-2 teaspoonfuls with warm water in the morning. You can also powder the black seed and mix with raw organic honey. For oil, take half a teaspoon in warm water.

It can help with joint pains, arthritis, stomach issues, kidney pain and infection, headaches, hair loss, skin diseases, dental diseases, anaemia, cough, constipation, and sleeplessness.

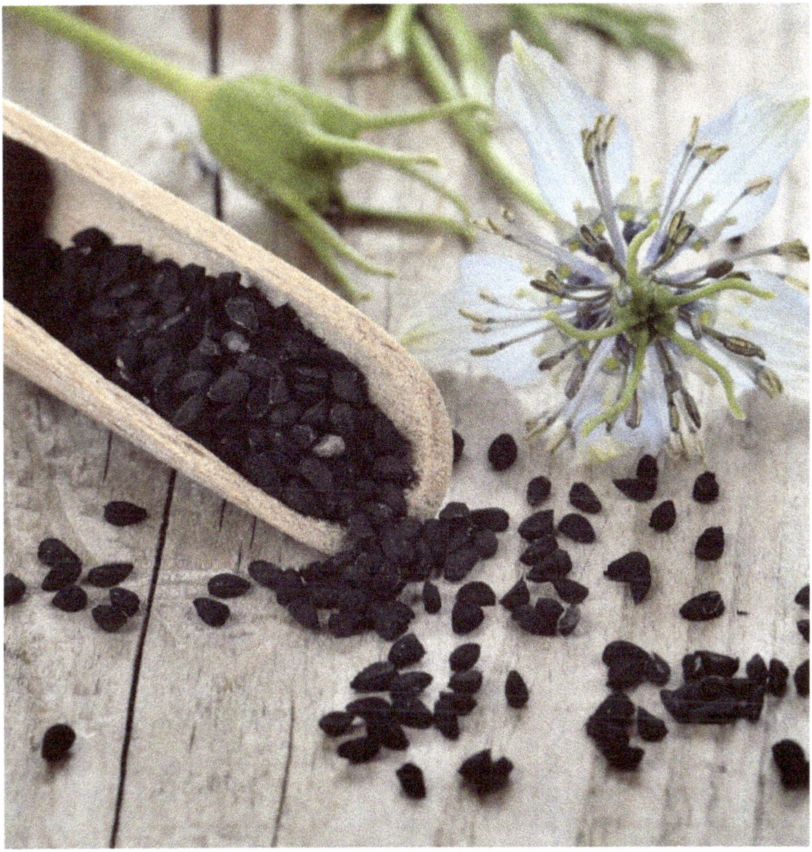

Honey – The Complete Food and Remedy

> "... *there issues from within their bodies a drink of varying colours, wherein is healing for men, verily, in this is a Sign for those who give thought.*"
>
> (Sūrah an-Naḥl, āyah 69)

Since ancient times, honey has been used as a food, medicine, and beauty enhancer. The earliest recorded medicinal uses date back to Sumerian tablets from around 1900 B.C.E. where it was used in up to 30% of prescriptions. It was a common remedy in Ancient Egypt for diseases of the eyes and skin. In Greece, it was used to prevent fatigue, and Hippocrates considered it an excellent cough expectorant. Honey has also been widely used in Europe, Arabia, and China as a remedy for gastric and intestinal complaints.

Honey's main constituents are bee pollen, propolis, and royal jelly. Bee pollen is a complete protein with essential amino acids, vitamins, minerals, and antioxidant-rich flavonoids. Propolis is rich in vitamins B-complex, C, E, and pro-vitamin A. Royal jelly, exclusive food for the queen bee, contains water, protein, carbohydrates, lipids, and vitamins B1, B2, B6, niacin, pantothenic acid, folic acid, and trace amounts of vitamin C.

The use of honey can help energy and mental alertness in children. A pre-bedtime teaspoon of honey can help address bedwetting.

Honey serves as a gentle remedy for constipation. Honey in barley water can alleviate stomach upsets. A mix of honey and cinnamon in hot water can provide relief for cold and cough. Honey and saffron in warm milk, before bed, can promote better sleep.

Honey is a natural antiseptic that can be applied on minor burns, bruises and cuts. A blend of honey and olive oil can be applied to the hair for improved lustre. Honey, oatmeal, and rose water create a complexion-enhancing facial suitable for all skin types. Honey mixed with beaten egg white is beneficial for oily skin or with milk cream for dry skin. Honey in bath water can alleviate fatigue.

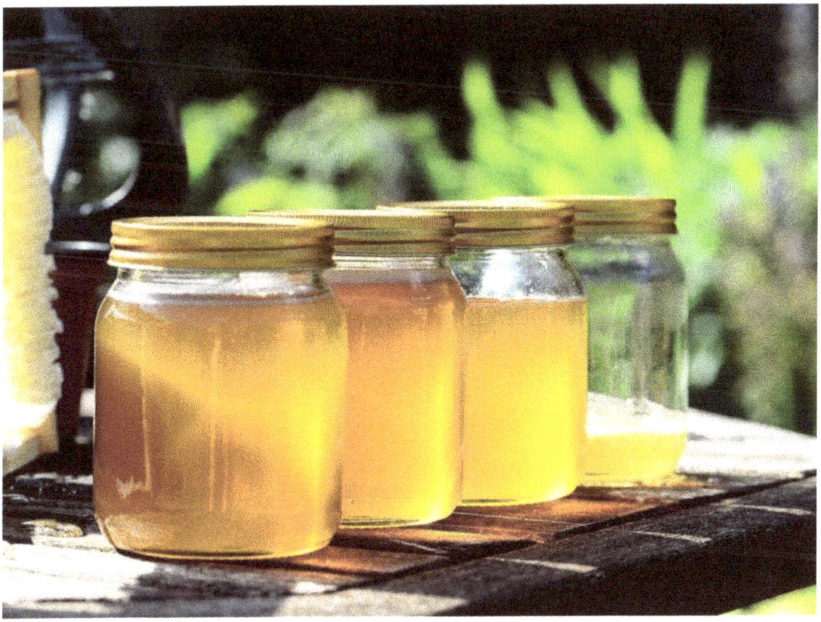

INDEX

A

Abbasid, 16-20
ʿAbd al-Laṭīf al-Baghdādī, 21
ʿAbd ar-Raḥīm ad-Dakhwar, 21
Abū'l-ʿAbbās ʿAbdullah as-Saffāḥ, 16
Abū'l-Qāsim az-Zahrāwī, 15
Abū ʿAlī ibn Sīnā, *see* Ibn Sīnā
Abū Bakr ibn Samghūn, 14
Abū Ḥāmid Muḥammad as-Samarqandī, 21
Abū ʿImrān Mūsā ibn Maymūn, *see* Maimonides
Abū Jaʿfar (al-Mansūr), *see* al-Mansūr
Abū Marwān ibn Zuhr, 16
Abū'l-Ḥasan al-Andalūsī, 14
Aʿḍā, 52-3
ad-dunyā, 34
Adnān, 4
Ahwaz, 18
air, 41-5, 47, 57-8, 62, 73
Akhlāt, *see* Humours
al-Ākhirah, 34
alchemy, 13, 20
ad-Dakhwar, *see* ʿAbd ar-Raḥīm ad-Dakhwar
ʿAlā' ad-Dīn ibn Nafīs, *see* Ibn Nafīs
Alexandrain, 19
al-Ghazālī, 98
al-Ḥāwī, 20
al-Ḥijāz, 4, 62
ʿAlī, 12
ʿAlī ibn Rabban aṭ-Ṭabarī, *see* aṭ-Ṭabarī
al-Mansūr, 17-8
al-Qānūn fi'ṭ-Ṭibb, 20
ʿamal ṣulḥah, 10
amānah, 31
Anatolia, 22
anatomy, 53-4
Andalusia, 14, 16
anus, 78
ʿaql, 40, 104
Aqrabadin, 96, 104
Arabia, pre-Islamic: alcohol, 6; health, 2, 6; promiscuity, 5; tribal chauvinism, 5; women's status, 5-6
Arabian Peninsula, 2, 117
Arkān, 42, 104, *see also* Elements
arteries, 51, 53-4, 57
aṭ-Ṭabarī, 19
āyah, 104, 110
Aydinolu Umar Bey, 22
Ayurvedic physicians, 23

B

Baghdad, 17-21, 104
Bangladesh, 101
Bayt al-Ḥikmah, 18-9, 104
Bile, see 'Yellow Bile'
Bimaristān, 17
Black Bile (Humour), 45-6, 51, 59, 74-5, 104, 108
bladder, 47, 84
Blood (Humour), 45, 47, 59, 69, 75, 104
bones, 29, 31, 46, 51, 53

bowels, 84, 95
brain, 29, 39-40, 47, 53-4, 82, 95, 107
Bukht Yishu, 18
Bulghum, 45, 47, 105, *see also* Phlegm
burial, 86

C

Cairo, 21
capillaries, 48
cauterisation, 7, 10
civilisation, 2, 4, 19
cognition, 39-40
conation, 39
consciousness, 31, 34, 39, 67, 78, 80, 87, 90, 108
Cordoba, 14-15, 21
cosmology, 41
cosmos, 27-29, 33, 41

D

Damascus, 17, 22
Dār al-Funūn, 21
Daʿwah, 94
decoctions, 93
Dīn-I-Fiṭra, 27
delirium, 67
Dhakhīrah Y Khwarzam, 21
diagnosis, 30, 36, 49, 52, 65, 68, 71, 74, 102
diet, 56-7, 90-1; consciousness, 90; emotions, 90
disease, classification, 66-8; definition, 66; functional, 67; spiritual, 67; structural, 68 superficial, 68
Dum, *see* Blood

E

Earth (Element), 41-43, 45
Egypt, 4, 7, 13, 18, 21, 22
electuaries, 93
Elements, 29, 41-48, 49, 53, 104
elixirs, 93
embryo, 38
energy, 41-2, 45, 90-1, 93-4, 107
exercise, effects, 81-2; physical, 80; prophylactic, 80; varieties, 81-2
eye, diseases, 6, 59; operations, 99; strengthening, 83; works, 19

F

faculty, attractive, 47; digestive, 37, 47; expulsive, 38, 47, 59; formative, 38; generative, 38; individuation, 37
Fajr (prayer time), 78
fasting, 87-88
Fatimids, 21
Firdaws al Ḥikmah, 19
Fire (Element), 41, 42, 44, 45, 47, 104, 108
fisq, 10
folk, medicine, 7; tradition, 90
food, *see* diet
frankincense, 4, 110

G

Galen, 19
gall-bladder, 48
garlic, 87
ghā'ib, 29, 39
Ghusl, 85
Granada, 14
Greece, 4, 7, 18

Greek, scholars, 13; works, 13, 19, 96
Gulf, of Aden, 2; of Oman, 2; Persian, 2

H

Hae Pasha, Ḥakīm, 22
Ḥajjāj ibn Yūsuf, 14
Ḥakīm, 22-3, 33, 56, 90, 96-7, 99, 101, 105, 112, 115-118
Hulagu, 20
ḥalāl, 10, 105
ḥammām, 85
health, definition, 32; essentials, 56; indications, 65-66; prevention, 78-88
hearing, 39, 83
heart, 34-5, 37, 40, 48, 51, 53-4, 71, 85, 89, 95, 107
ḥifẓ aṣ-ṣiḥḥah, 86
Ḥijāz, 4, 62
Hippocrates, 19
human being, 1, 10, 26-32, 34, 36-7, 41-2, 48, 65, 89, 92, 97, 103-4, 108, 116
Humours, 36, 45-48, 58-9, 61-63, 72, 74-76, 90-1, 104-5, 108

I

ʿibādah, 32
Ibn Abī ʿUsaybiah, 21
Ibn al-Bayṭār, 14
Ibn Allahaj, 18
Ibn Bājah, 16
Ibn Masawayh, 18-19
Ibn Nafīs, 21, 99
Ibn Qurrah, 19
Ibn Rushd, 16
Ibn Sīnā, 20, 96, 113, 114
Ibn Ṭufayl, 16
Ibn Uthal, 13
ilhām, 39
India, 7, 18, 22, 23, 101, 117
infertility, 10
infusions, 93
insān, *see* human being
Iran, 18, 21, 22, *see also* Persia
Iraq, 17
Islamic medicine, economics, 102; future, 100-103; history, 2-23; philosophy, 24-33; physiology, 41-55; psychology, 34-40
iʿtidāl, 106

J

Jābir ibn Ḥayyan, 13
Jaʿfar aṣ-Ṣādiq, Imam 13
Jalāluddīn Rūmī, *see* Rūmī
Jibrīl Bukht Yishu, 18
Jinn, 4
jism, 34, 106
Jundishapur, 12, 17, 18
Jurjis ibn Bukht Yishu, *see* Bukht Yishu

K

Khālid bin Yazīd, 13
Khan, Muḥammad Ajmal, 23; Genghis, 22
Khwarzam, 21
Khilāfat ar-Rāshidah, 12-13
khamr, 6, 106
kidneys, 47, 51, 58, 74, 75, 95
Kitāb al-Aghdiyah, 16
Kitāb al-Asbāb wa'l-ʿAlāmāt, 21
Kitāb al-ʿAshr Maqālāt fi'l ʿAyn, 19
Kitāb al-Fuṣūl, 16
Kitāb at-Taṣrīf, 15, 98
Kitāb at-Taysīr fi'l-Mudāwāt Wa't-Tadbīr, 16

Kitāb Tadbīr aṣ-Ṣiḥḥah, 16

L

laṭīf, 36, 106
laws, 28, 36, 38, 54
leprosy, 6, 10
leucoderma, 38
liver, 37, 47, 51, 53, 54, 74, 75, 95, 107
lungs, 47, 51, 54, 57, 95

M

macrocosm, 29, 30, 42
magic, 8, 10, 97
Maimonides, 16, 21
Makkah, 5, 8-9, 63, 80
Malaga, 14
malaria, 6
Malaysia, 101
Mankha, 19
Masīḥ al-Mulk, *see* Khan, Muḥammad Ajmal
massage, 82, 84-5
Materia Medica, 14, 52, 96
medicine, European, 21-22; folk, 7; Islamic, *see* Islamic medicine; Prophetic, *see* Ṭibb, an-Nabawī; *see also* Ṭibb
Madinah, 9, 11
Mediterranean, 3
memory, 40, 65, 82
microcosm, 29-31, 42
miswāk, 79, 106
mizāj, 48, 51, 107, *see also* temperament
Mu'āwiyah, 13
mufradāt, 92, 106
Muhammad ﷺ, 1, 2, 7-12, 16, 89
Muḥammad Ḥasan, Ḥakīm, 23
Muhammad ibn Zakariyyā ar-Rāzī, *see* Rāzī
murakkabāt, 92, 108
myrrh, 4, 110

N

nafs, 30, 34-5, 107; al-ammārah, 35; al–muṭma'innah, 35; al-lawwāmah, 35
nerves, 29, 39, 51, 53-4

O

onions, 4, 87
organs, 6, 26, 30, 37, 39, 45-48, 50-54, 68, 74, 80-1, 83, 87, 93, 95
ovaries, 37, 54, 108

P

Pakistan, 22-3, 101, 117
pathology, 36
penis, 54
perfumes, 5, 87
Persia, 7, 12, 18, 20
Persian, Gulf, 2; language, 22
pharmaceutical, 102
pharmacognosy, 92
philosophy, 27, 31, 32, 97
Phlegm (Humour), 45, 47, 50-1, 59, 75, 104-5
physiological concepts, 41, 55
pills, 93
plague, 86
prevention, 27, 78, 106
psychology, 34, 40
puberty, 58, 88
pulse, 71-73, 75

Q

qalb, 34, 89, 107 *see also* heart
Qaḥṭān, 4
qiblah, 80
Quraysh, 3, 9, 13
Qu'rān, 1, 8-10, 61, 98
quwwah, 41-2, 114, *see also* energy
quwwah an-nāṭiqiyah, 39
quwwah al-mutafakkirah, 39
quwwah al-mughayarah, 37

R

Rāzī, 17, 20, 96
rectum, 48
Red Sea, 2
renaissance, 26
rest, 31, 41, 43, 56, 63, 84-85
retention, 56, 64
Rey (in Persia), 20
rickets, 6
rīḥ, 82
Rubʿ al-Khālī, 3
rūh, 35-36; definition, 107; ḥaywāniyyah, 37; nafsāniyyah, 39; ṭabayyah, 37; *see also* vital force
Rūmī, 24-25
ruqyā, 98

S

Saffavid, 21
Ṣafrā, *see* Yellow Bile
ṣaḥīḥah, 32
sakīnah, 32, 108
Ṣalāh, 79-80
Ṣalāḥuddīn, 17
salīmah, 32
salivation, 70
Samarqand, 19, 21, 65
Saudā, *see* Black Bile
Ṣawm, *see* fasting
schizophrenia, 67
scurvy, 6
semen, 38
Shahādah, 28
Shamals, 4
Shams-i-Tabrīzī, 41
Sharīʿah, 97, 108, 116
Shifā' al-Mulk, *see* Muḥammad Ḥasan, Ḥakīm
siḥr, *see* magic
sleep, 30, 56, 61, 65, 70, 85
smallpox, 22
smell, 39, 47, 74-5
Spain, 14-16, 21
spleen, 45-6, 51, 74-5
stomach, 45-6, 54, 68-9, 71, 85, 94-5, 107
stool, 58, 75-77
suicide, 67
sulphur, 63
surgery, 15-16, 98-99, 117
Syria, 2, 5, 18

T

Ṭabīb, 101; al-Kāmil, 1
tablets, 93
ṭahārah, 86, 108
Tā'if, 3
tanwīn, 99
taqwā, 87, 108
taste, 37, 46, 61, 68
ṭayyib, 10, 62
Tehran, 21
temperament, 48-52, 84, 89, 94, 115; age, 50; balanced, 65; cold, 70; definition, 48; dry, 70-1; females, 50; hot, 69; medicines,

51-2; organs, 50-1, signs, 68-71; *see also* mizāj
temperature, 4, 39, 57, 72
testicles, 36, 51, 102
Thābit ibn Qurrah, *see* Ibn Qurrah
Ṭibb, 1, 66, 89, 96, 109; al-Islāmī, 32; an-Nabawī, 1, 109
Tigris, 17
tinctures, 93
touch, 39, 70
tuberculosis, 6
Turkey, 22

U

'Umar, 12
Umayyad, 13-17
ummah, 86
unity, 27-29, 32-36, 40-41, 55, 66
urine, 58, 70, 74-76
uterus, 54

V

veins, 51, 54, 83
Vienna, 22
vision, 39
vital force, 35-39, 45, 51, 57, 59, 60, 71-73, 91, 107, *see also* 'rūh'

W

waḥi, 7, 27, 109
Walīd ibn 'Abd al-Malik, 13
Water (Element), 41, 43-45, 47, 104-105.
water, 42, 47, 57-58, 62-63, 83, 86; purification with, 78-79; zamzam, see 'zamzam'
wisdom, 2, 18, 24, 33, 38, 78,103-5
womb, *see* uterus
wuḍū', 79

X

xerophytic, 4

Y

Yellow Bile (Humour), 45, 47-48, 50, 59-60, 69, 75-76, 104, 108
Yemen, 5
Yuhanna ibn Masawayh, *see* Ibn Masawayh

Z

ẓāhir, 29, 39
zamzam (water), 114
Zayn ad-Dīn Islmā'īl al-Ḥusaynī al Jurjānī, 21
zinc, 63

About the Author

M. Salim Khan M.D. (M.A.) M.H. D.O. is an international authority on natural medicine known especially for his person-centred, wisdom-based practice of Tibb, naturopathy, herbal medicine, nutrition, iridology, counselling, and psychotherapy.

M. Salim Khan has been in practice since 1978. His teachers and inspirations in Tibb include Shabeer Hussain Sahib (ra), Moulana Nisaar Ahmed (ra) and Hakim Nabi Khan Sahib (ra). He trained in herbal medicine and osteopathy with the General Council and Register of Consultant Medical Herbalists (now IRCH). He studied iridology and nutrition with Dr. B. C. Jensen and Farida Sharan. He taught nutrition and iridology at the School of Iridology and Wholistic Healing, Cambridge, England.

At the time of publication, M. Salim Khan is the president of the Guild of Naturopathic Iridologists International (GNI) and The Guild of Unani Tibb (TGU). He is also a trustee of the World Unani Foundation (WUF). He is the director of Mohsin Health Clinic, Products and Publications based in Leicester, UK, and the Principal of the College of Medicine and Healing Arts (CoMHA).

M. Salim Khan's other books include *The Golden Key to Discovering Yourself*, which offers a more detailed look into the Tibb understanding of temperaments in relation to health.

Learn More About Tibb

The College of Medicine and Healing Arts (CoMHA) is led by M. Salim Khan, registered in England and Wales as a not-for-profit. The underlying philosophy is one of inclusiveness, seeing unity in diversity. The training and education provided by the College of Medicine and Healing Arts is authentically rooted in the Tibb tradition, provided in holistic traditional practices, integrating modern knowledge and skills where appropriate. Based in Leicester, England, United Kingdom, the College facilitates professional in-person training programmes in the UK and worldwide.

Graduates of the College's professional Diploma courses are able to run safe, effective, legal, ethical, and financially sustainable professional practices as naturopaths and herbalists, or as counsellors and psychotherapists. Graduates will be able to safely and competently help patients and clients, with a focus on preventing and recovering from diseases of contemporary modern life.

For the public, the College offers free educational articles and videos on its website. In-person weekends, retreats, and workshops are available for personal benefit, as well as online courses.

Visit **www.CoMHA.org.uk** to access free educational resources as well as learn more about all the courses currently being offered.

www.ingramcontent.com/pod-product-compliance
Lightning Source LLC
Chambersburg PA
CBHW042130160426
43198CB00022B/2961
* 9 7 8 0 9 9 2 9 4 5 6 2 6 *